HEALING PEOPLE, NOT PATIENTS

Creating Authentic Relationships in Modern Healthcare

Jonathan Weinkle, MD

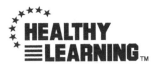

HEALTHY LEARNING™

ISBN: 978-1-60679-440-1
Library of Congress Control Number: 2018953114
Book layout: Cheery Sugabo
Cover design: Cheery Sugabo

Healthy Learning
P.O. Box 1828
Monterey, CA 93942
www.healthylearning.com

This book was made possible through the generous support of the Jewish Healthcare Foundation.

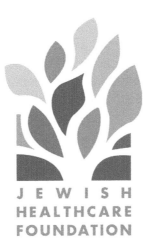

The Jewish Healthcare Foundation (JHF) is a nonprofit public charity that was established in 1990 with proceeds from the sale of Montefiore Hospital, a healthcare institution financed and founded by Pittsburgh's Jewish community. JHF and its three operating arms—the Pittsburgh Regional Health Initiative (PRHI), Health Careers Futures (HCF), and the Women's Health Activist Movement Global (WHAMglobal)—develop and manage programs, conduct research and training, and make grants to perfect patient care. JHF is also the fiscal agent for state HIV/AIDS funding in southwestern Pennsylvania.

DEDICATION

This book is dedicated to my mentor-from-afar, Bernard Lown, MD. I discovered his book *The Lost Art of Healing* in the back of a Half Price Books in the summer of 2000 and it became the mission statement for my career in medicine. While we have never met, I constantly feel his hand guiding mine as I try to do right by the people I care for. May my own modest work be a step toward ensuring that the art of healing is no longer lost.

ACKNOWLEDGMENTS

I've read many books since finishing this manuscript, most of them by people who endured tremendous suffering to earn the insight that made their books worth writing (and reading). Basic training and residency were walks in the park by comparison; I have come through life relatively unscathed and blessed. That, and this book, are thanks to the following people.

The Jewish Healthcare Foundation, and especially Nancy Zionts and Karen Wolk Feinstein. Years ago, when I first conceived of this book in the form of a 20-page independent study during my second year of medical school, Nancy read it, loved it, and believed that somewhere along the line it would find its way to light. Without the support of JHF, it would likely still be no more than a paper in my filing cabinet. Without Karen's deep reading and extensive critiques of three full drafts of the manuscript, it would likely still be all over the map and drowning in pedantic footnotes. Thanks to them, it is exactly what I dreamed it would be, even when I didn't really understand the dream.

The health center, for being so thoughtful as to open for business and create my dream job for me down the street from my house just as I was finishing residency. Thank you especially to Susan Friedberg Kalson and Andrea Fox, for hiring me, for giving me the opportunity to care for such wonderful people, and for green-lighting this project so we could share our philosophy of care with the world.

Speaking of the health center, the nurses, medical assistants, therapists, nurse practitioners, doctors, physician assistants, front desk staff, social workers, and dental at a place that might as well adopt the motto of the 4077th *M*A*S*H*—"Best Care Anywhere." Right, Radar?

My mentors and colleagues who taught me things I had to pass on in these pages, who showed me a better way to care for people, and who rolled up their sleeves when I needed help giving someone the care they deserved. I will forget someone for sure, but: Rabbi Larry Heimer, Rabbi Eli Seidman, Rabbi Nosson Sacks, Father Sam Esposito, Daniel Leger, Pastor Richard Freeman, Rabbi Ron Symons, Rabbi Danny Schiff, Rabbi Mike Werbow, Russ Kolarik, Sylvia Choi, Dena Hofkosh, Bill Cohen, Ev Vogeley, Karen Barnard, Bob Arnold, Gary Fischer, Nathan Bahary, Noam Gilboa, Thuy Buy, Stuart Fisk, Alda Maria Gonzaga, Maxim Hammer, Robin Girdhar, Elana Bloom, Susan Hunt, Melanie Gold, Mike Wollman, Matt Schuchert, Jessica Perini, Scott Tyson, Devra Davis, Sanjay Lambore, Natalia Morone, and Reed Van Deusen.

The "village" of Squirrel Hill (as in "It takes a village"), for supporting me through this project, spying on my children so they wouldn't get in trouble, and exemplifying how we ought to care for people when they are ill, sad, or overwhelmed by the joy and exhaustion of a new baby. Special thanks to longtime villager Danny Rosen for insisting that people *had* to read what I had written.

Speaking of the village, Ilana Schwarcz, for being an excellent (and fast!) editor. It was a pleasure working with you—and a greater pleasure to have your family as our friends.

Jim Peterson and Kristi Huelsing from Healthy Learning, for taking a flyer on a book by a first-time author. Thank you for believing in me and giving me the chance to take this mission to the next stage.

Deborah Gilboa, aka Dr. G from the *Today* show, who sits at the desk next to me, punches me in the arm, provides witty quotes for this book, and makes me a better doctor. We joked about working together when our oldest kids were toddlers, and someone built us a health center. Never hurts to ask.

The "framily" that started when Ari Gilboa and Eitan Weinkle were 11 months old and didn't know that children their age weren't supposed to play interactively, and that now sustains all of us from Friday to Friday and through the whole mess in between.

My in-laws, Lia and Natan Nemirovsky. The wisdom of their immigrant experience and the warmth of their home has opened my mind and my heart to be so much more than my neat, linear American self could have otherwise been.

My boys, Eitan, Akiva, and Adi. You have taken the gentle pushes, nudges, leading by example, love, and benign neglect and become exactly the people Mom and I hoped you would.

My parents, Phyllis and Joe Weinkle, who are wise, sensible, caring, and supportive. I think I inherited those last two qualities because I just wrote a book about using them in the clinic; the jury is still out on the first two.

And most of all, my wife, Vita Nemirovsky, who took the raw material my parents handed her and made me into the person I am today—without her I would not have been capable of the insight that I needed to write this book or live by its message.

CONTENTS

INTRODUCTION: MORE THAN AN ADVENTURE

The US military used to recruit with TV commercials that promised aspiring soldiers, "It's not just a job—it's an adventure."

Practicing medicine is not just a job either, and boy, can it be an adventure. But in my experience, it is not "just an adventure." Practicing medicine is a privilege, a gift—a sacred trust.

This book is about how to make the day-to-day practice of medicine reflect that sacredness, even when internal and external forces drag doctors and patients away from the trusting relationship between two human beings and into the mundane, or even the profane. It is about how to ensure that the fundamental building block of that relationship, the face-to-face encounter between one who seeks healing and one who heals, benefits from open, honest communication, mutual respect, and shared purpose, even when systemic problems push them into adversarial positions.

I've been fortunate enough to practice for 10 years and counting in a Federally Qualified Health Center whose only mission is to provide this kind of care and do so at the highest possible level of quality, for a group of patients as diverse and varied— and fascinating—as humanity itself. In a way, I am writing to share my feeling that the approach to healthcare we are continuing to develop within our walls is the kind of care that all people in need of healing deserve, even as we strive to get even better at what we do.

From those eight years, and the nine years of training that preceded them, I have accumulated a lot of stories. These stories bring urgency and immediacy to what I want to say about the practice of medicine. Legally and morally, however, telling stories is a tricky business. Modern medicine jealously protects patient privacy and confidentiality, so much that even revealing that I am someone's doctor to a third party without their permission is a violation of the law. But the tradition of guarding privacy goes back further than that, as is necessary in a profession where people often reveal their innermost secrets, under the assumption that nothing leaves the room without permission. Those secrets, once revealed, still belong to the teller, not the hearer. As a result, these fascinating stories, strictly speaking, are not mine to tell, except insofar as I was present and insofar as *I changed or grew* in being part of the hearing.

The stories you read, therefore, are true in the sense that everything in them happened *to me*—but it may have happened to a composite of several different patients, or it may have happened to one person, whose identity I have deliberately obfuscated by changing identifying details. My CEO once remarked that she sometimes shares success stories with our funders that have been so carefully reworked that the doctor who told her the story doesn't even recognize the episode. I have hoped to veil my stories just as well that the patients might not recognize *themselves,* other than through a sort of universal empathy.

In the interest of a compelling story, I have tried to streamline the narrative by keeping the footnotes and citations to a minimum, but clearly any work like this stands on many shoulders. For those interested in reading the lay and medical literature that underpins much of what I have to say, I have included an extensive bibliography. The specific sources for facts and quotes in each chapter are summarized in the "Notes" section at the end of the book.

The book also draws heavily on my reading of Jewish sources. I have called the relationship between seeker and healer a sacred trust, and for me personally sacred and Jewish are equivalent terms. For as long as I have studied medicine, I have studied in parallel to figure out not just how to do it well, but how to do it in a holy manner, consistent with my beliefs. Yet, I recognize that this is a call to physicians of all faiths, or of no faith at all, to practice a medicine that is singularly devoted to the unique human being in need of healing, and that the modern Hippocratic Oath calls for us to swear by "what each of us holds most sacred." Therefore, you can read the narrative as it is, and know that my sacred sources are bubbling beneath the surface, without having to read, recognize, or buy into them. I have, however, included an appendix so that those who are interested in traveling down that deep well can study the texts and traditions I have drawn from in building each chapter.

Let's begin our adventure—and so much more.

CHAPTER 1
Pedestal

My middle child once came home from pre-school and declared his science teacher "almost as smart as God." When we told the teacher this, she was pleasantly amused, as were we. Then, this happened to me:

A tiny woman from South Asia, dressed elegantly in layers of gold-and-burgundy cloth, with several strands of beads on her neck and intricate earrings framing both ears, sat nearly silently before me for the better part of 30 minutes. She had waved away my offer of a professional phone interpreter, gesturing instead toward her son. He was a man my own age, with a Western college education, fluent colloquial English, and a thoroughly American style of dress. He answered many of my questions to her, without even bothering to translate. When I did insist that he question her directly instead of presuming to answer for her, her replies were sparse, perhaps two or three words, followed by a long pause, in which she looked expectantly back toward her son to pick up the thread of the conversation.

She asked no questions of her own, despite my regular asides to check in with her for understanding. I examined her thoroughly, often needing to repeat or rephrase instructions two or three times. In 70 years on Earth, she might have seen a doctor five times and hadn't developed the automatic behaviors of breathing deeply, relaxing to have her reflexes checked, or lying flat on her back (instead of curled on her side) to have her abdomen examined. Through all of this, she remained nearly mute.

As I completed my instructions to the woman's son, I felt a heavy disappointment. I teach my students the maxim, "Nothing about me, without me," a mantra from the disability advocacy movement that means, "Hey, I'm a real person—don't discuss my affairs or my medical care as if I'm not in the room." Yet, here I had just completed a comprehensive health visit, in which the person ostensibly at the center had been almost a bystander—a model or museum exhibit of an actual person who was not really present. Somehow, I had failed her.

At that moment, my patient spoke. Not loudly, but slowly, quietly, and not to anyone in particular. She nodded and smiled as she did, speaking in a steady cadence for a couple of minutes, longer than she had spoken for the entire visit to that point put together. I followed none of the words, having no common language that even resembled what she was speaking, but I remember listening intently to every sound she made, as if expecting her to suddenly switch into English, or Spanish, or some other language I might recognize.

When she finished, she sat back and folded her arms and beamed, and now it was my turn to expectantly turn toward her son.

"She says thank you. She says you are our family doctor, and you have helped us so much and I am very grateful for all your help. In our culture, the doctor is next to the God."

There were a thousand things I could have said in reply, and all of them were wrong, either too arrogant, or too self-deprecating, or too flippant. I could also have said nothing—and failed to acknowledge the only words this woman had said out loud the whole visit. In the end, I think I mumbled something underwhelming enough that I don't remember it at all, and moved on from this important moment, as if the woman had been commenting on the weather. "Yes, it's raining, what of it?"

So, God tested me again, and I soon found myself dealing with versions of this conversation as a recurring theme, perhaps half a dozen times over the next few months. I was going to need a good answer.

It's not as though I couldn't have seen this moment coming. Growing up, from the middle of high school to the end of college, I was planning a career as a congregational rabbi—and was told in not so many words, "What kind of job is that for a nice Jewish boy?" It wasn't because these well-meaning adults had any bias against the rabbinate; it was because they wanted me to be a doctor. Forget about me—I actually know a *rabbi* who told his son, now *also* a rabbi—that he could choose any career he wanted, after he was done with medical school. The greatest Jewish mind of the past 1800 years, Moses Maimonides? Sure, he was a rabbi and an astronomer and a philosopher—but he was also the greatest doctor of his generation.

Doctors live on a pedestal. They save us the prime parking spots in the garage and a private cafeteria in the hospital. We can dodge speeding tickets and get out of jury duty. Jewish doctors, like me, are allowed, under religious law, to dispense with Sabbath observance, laws of physical modesty, and even release people from fasting on Yom Kippur, if it's necessary to save a life. We've been getting *carte blanche* across cultures and through the centuries.

It seems almost too obvious to even ask why. Doctors save lives, or so we allow the public to believe. We seem to be the one thing that can stand between them and the inevitability of death, at least for a little while. Making a deal with the doctor seems like a better alternative than making a deal with the devil …

But for many years, that wasn't the pedestal I wanted to stand on. Like most teenagers, I was not about to go quietly into the good night of adulthood, doing exactly what was expected of me. The fact that my rebellion consisted of wanting to be a rabbi tells you how lousy I was at teenage rebellion. But, the fact is, I didn't care about the prestige, the income, or that "everybody knew" that smart kids went to med school. I was interested in "big ideas," things that transcended the everyday: faith, symbolism, music, prayer, and ultimate meaning. I didn't choose to major in biochemistry in college, I majored in philosophy. I was looking for a life where I touched people's lives through sermons, not syringes, and where I lived my Jewishness every minute.

I wouldn't say I hated science at that stage, but I think I believed it was cold and inhuman; I had read too much dystopian science fiction. But strangely, as I went through my philosophy classes, it was the ones that grappled with the philosophy of science, and even the one "straight" science class I took, biology, that made the biggest impact on me. Some of my philosophy classes, the ones on rationalism and empiricism, in particular, left me colder emotionally than high school chemistry had done. But, the classes that dealt with the nexus of science, religion, and philosophy were the ones that brought me to life. They were asking the questions I really cared about: What were miracles, really? How "true" were scientific discoveries, and were they more "true" than religious truth, or just different? Was there a single "reality," or multiple viewpoints that could never be fully intelligible to one another? Could science tell us the right way for people to treat one another—or was that a question only faith could answer?

I graduated with the degree in philosophy, unemployable and not really sure any longer what I wanted to do with it. And now, there was the new interest in the sciences, a sensation I hadn't felt since grade school, when I was rereading astronomy books every night. A career in astronomy, or chemistry, or engineering, didn't fit. I didn't want to spend my time in a lab, or doing field research, or working with machinery. I wanted people: daily, deep human interactions, the kind of relationships that drew me into the rabbinate before this. Maybe medicine after all? Maybe the adults in my life had seen this about me when I couldn't, that it was the one way to get my brain involved with the hard sciences, while keeping my heart focused on the "soft" truth of meaning and emotion.

About the same time as I came to this conclusion, I had entered my military service in the Israel Defense Forces Naval Corps. I was a medic, the equivalent of a hospital corpsman in the US military. One of the first thoughts I had after I finished training and started staffing the daily sick call was, "This is interesting as far as it goes, but I can't spend the rest of my life handing out Tums and Tylenol." I was also hoping never to use my combat lifesaving training. I eventually did, once, but it was to save a fisherman who nearly drowned, trying to fish from a boulder 500 meters from shore, not under fire. I wasn't on a pedestal—I was at the very bottom of a totem pole. All the same, I was intrigued at what life was like at the top of that pole.

What was strange is that even in that role, people showed me some amount of deference. I spent about a week in a remote outpost toward the end of my first summer in the service. I probably saw 10 soldiers for various minor complaints during that time, and then returned to my own base the following week. One morning, a radar operator I had taken care of during that week posting showed up at the main base— and handed me a sunflower she had picked on the side of the road. "For listening to me last week and not being a jerk," she told me. Not for getting the diagnosis right, not for getting her out of duty, but just for listening.

I remembered something I had been told by a friend, while working at summer camp during college. "You have this face that makes me feel like I could tell you anything." I had often viewed this as a mixed blessing, as I have a tendency to attract strangers on buses and airplanes, who readily shared their entire life stories, their sometimes uncomfortable political opinions, and their earnest career advice. Now, I was beginning to think this would come in handy.

Healing People, Not Patients

Maybe a month or two later, my friend Assaf, a very tall, lanky guy who worked as a shipyard mechanic, came into the infirmary, with his left hand wrapped in a bloody rag. He was stooped over, looking anxious and guilty.

"I was in the shop after breakfast working on an outboard motor for one of the lifeboats and my hand got caught—not even really sure between what and what. All I know is the pain was intense, like fire, and there was blood everywhere. My commander wrapped it in the first rag he could find and brought me over here."

I cringed; only a few weeks had passed since one of our best ship's engineers had lost two fingers in his engine, and a good bit of his identity as a sailor along with it. He went from a gregarious jokester to an angry, bitter, gloomy person overnight. Now, I was afraid I was about to untie the rag and see history in the process of repeating itself with Assaf.

At first blush, I was relieved—everything still attached, no exposed tendons, just messy, mangled skin and some rapidly clotting, drying blood. His fingers moved easily, though he grimaced as they did so, and his nails were still pink, and his fingertips warm. The hand would survive. I was just about to look up and tell him the good news before cleaning him up and taking him over to the doctor's office, when Assaf leaned in to me and whispered to me in a conspiratorial tone, "I know why this happened."

"Why's that?" I answered without looking up. I was still trying to figure out the best way to clean his hand off, without putting him through horrible agony, so I was staring into the wound, instead of looking him in the eye.

"It's because I didn't put on *tefillin* this morning," he said glumly.

I knew Assaf was a deeply religious guy; most mornings he made a beeline from the gate of the base to the synagogue for the morning service before commencing his work. Apparently, today, he was late, and afraid of getting in trouble, so he bypassed the synagogue and went straight to the shop. Missing services meant he also skipped putting on *tefillin*, leather boxes containing passages from the Torah that are strapped to the arm and forehead to remind a person to fix the words of God in front of his eyes and bind them tightly to his every action. As a right-handed person, he would have put these on his left arm, wrapped in such a way that the black leather straps would wind around his palm in a crow's foot pattern and then snake up his fingers—right over the spots that were now oozing blood.

I'd had my share of conversations like this before. As an American-born Conservative Jew, I was much more of a religious rationalist than many of my traditional Israeli friends who took a much more supernatural, mystical view of God. This led to a lot of arguments and insinuations that I was some kind of heretic. But, this was different; Assaf was in pain, and also in a lot of mental anguish over what he believed was divine retribution. Arguing with him didn't seem like the right thing to do in this situation.

I clapped him on the shoulder of his uninjured arm and stood, so I could face him from slightly above his eye level. "I don't think God works that way, brother. And *I* definitely don't think this is your fault. Let's go see the doctor."

"Thanks, Yoni, but I don't know. We'll see what happens. I sure don't plan to forget my *tefillin* again."

I'd be lying if I said this conversation was what made me decide I wanted to go into medicine after all. But looking back, it was definitely the first time I was consciously aware that by entering into a healing relationship with someone (even if I was the low man on the totem pole at the time) didn't just mean treating the bumps and bruises, stopping the bleeding, or securing an airway. It was the first time I recognized the existence of a deeper level of conversation, an existential meaning to what went on in the treatment room. What I had been looking for in the rabbinate turned out to exist in medicine, too. I decided to start climbing onto the pedestal after all.

Once I was in medical school, however, I realized that finding room for the meaning was hard, even in the most "human" science, medicine. Gross anatomy hits lead-off in the "batting order" of punishingly difficult courses in the first year. This means that the first "patient" most students encounter is dead, embalmed, and shortly thereafter in pieces—as well as a frequent subject of tasteless, uncomfortable jokes. Following anatomy, there are courses in biochemistry, cell biology, physiology (the study of the normal workings of the body), pathology (the study of disease), pathophysiology (the study of what happens when pathology and physiology collide, and the normal workings become abnormal), microbiology, pharmacology, and genetics.

About 2/3 of the way through first year, we began to take hybrid courses, based around the different organ systems of the body. There was a course on the heart, another on the lungs, and another on the gastrointestinal tract. This leads to some interesting anatomical questions (to which system does the mouth belong?) and some interesting approaches to disease (is diabetes a disease of the gastrointestinal tract, since it takes place in the liver and pancreas, or is it a hormonal disease that should be studied in the endocrinology block?).

This curriculum accurately reflects the way modern medicine focuses on the minutest parts of the body. The degree of minuteness increases with each passing year. Ophthalmologists are known for knowing everything there is to know about a part of the body that is less than one cubic inch. I have a friend who is a retina specialist, so he only deals with the back wall of that one cubic inch.

A self-effacing orthopedic surgeon friend of mine recommended, "Never ask for general medical advice from anyone whose specialty begins with "O:" ophthalmology, otolaryngology (ear, nose, and throat), orthopedics, and obstetrics." His first day of residency, his chief went down the line of interns with a pair of trauma shears and cut off their stethoscopes midway down the tubing, so they wouldn't be tempted to actually *use* them.

One of my best friends rotated through a cardiac intensive care unit during residency. On rounds one morning, he was discussing the problems of a patient who had an infection, in addition to his heart troubles. The attending cardiologist stopped him, raising one finger in the air, and then motioned across his chest with his hands, as if to make a little frame around the heart. This was the cardiac ICU, and if there was a problem with an infection, the residents could clearly solve it themselves or call in an infectious disease specialist.

This didn't sit well with me at all. Healing was supposed to be complete healing, healing of the soul and healing of the body. It wasn't supposed to be tweaking the dials on different organ systems, so separate from one another that they may as well have been different people. And sometimes the focus wasn't even on individual organs, but on processes taking place at a molecular level so far removed from the human scale that I couldn't even recognize them as such. People didn't seem like people; everything was programmed into their genetic code, reduced to numbers. I was learning that there was no room for the soul in the medicine.

Even in psychiatry, "the doctoring of the soul," this reductionist approach holds sway. We manipulate the serotonin receptor, the dopamine receptor, and the norepinephrine receptor in the brain, so that we can relieve depression, quell anxiety, and quiet the voices in people's heads. This is as close to the soul as we get.

Psychiatrists, in most settings, no longer have couches, no longer ask people about their earliest memories of their mothers, and no longer sit silently for hours waiting for the patient to get to the point. My father-in-law, a psychiatrist who actually spends an unusually long time talking with most of his patients, once said to me, "Every time we discover something really good, the neurologists take it over." It was all about the brain, not the soul.

Until intern year. Every intern has a "first night on call" story. Mine was spent squeezing breath into the lungs of a very gray-looking premature baby, just delivered and not engaging in "lusty, vigorous crying." Her APGAR score was a 1 (normal babies are usually a nine, out of a possible 10, and nobody is supposed to get a 10). So, the first things past her newborn lips were not a breast or even a bottle but a metal laryngoscope and a plastic endotracheal tube, through which I spent the next five minutes squeezing air, and then color, and ultimately life into this tiny little girl.

Adam was created this way, with God breathing life into a body fashioned out of dust as gray and lifeless as that baby was before we pumped her pink with an Ambu bag. Breath is life, so much so that even in this era of life-saving technology and brain death criteria, a call from my answering service to alert me of a death still says "CTB"—ceased to breathe. Breath is soul, so much so that the two words in Hebrew are identical save for one vowel sound. And soul is the kiss of God, the thing that takes dust, matter, flesh—and turns them into something Divine.

Kurt Vonnegut used to say that he grew up expecting that by 1951, scientists would have photographed God in Technicolor—an actual image of God. It was a nice idea, but even though I came of age reading Vonnegut, I also grew up believing that making an actual image of God was idolatry, reducing the infinite and transcendent to the mundane and profane. There was no body of God to photograph; Moses couldn't look at the face of God, because God doesn't have a face. God has a mind, and a soul, and the breath God pushed through Adam's lips meant that Adam, and every human being from that point forward, carried the image of God's mind inside them.

Talk about a pedestal. Not only doctors, but *all* human beings, are "next to God," transient images of the Divine trying to live up to that awesome legacy. But how?

Next time you walk into the coffee shop, look the barista in the eye and instead of just ordering a drink, stop for a minute and reframe the encounter. The barista is not just a functionary placed there to unite you with your preferred form of hot caffeine, but a human being with a divine spark inside. So is the person that just cut you off in traffic, and the relative you've been feuding with for the past three years. And if you're a doctor, so is the patient in front of you.

We forget that pretty easily. It didn't take me long as a third-year medical student on the hospital wards to see the way people become patients. Patients become diseases, room numbers, and procedures: "The cystic on 7 has *burkholderia cepacia*." "3313 needs her pain meds." "I'm swamped today—I have three colonoscopies, one EGD, and a gastric emptying study. See if you can cancel the barium swallow and move the flex sig to next week." Families' faces flush red with anger when they hear the nurses flippantly call their father, "the cabbage." Even realizing that 'cabbage' is actually 'CABG' and refers to the man's Coronary Artery Bypass Graft surgery does not heal the wound of their relative becoming your surgical procedure and nothing more. Patients that make us uncomfortable become nicknames, names like GOMER, 'shake and bake,' or the especially odious (and bigoted) 'status Hispanicus.'

To combat this tendency, my medical school did something that at the time, in the late 1990s, was quite different, though it has become more common over time. I said that students' first patient was always dead and embalmed—but not ours. Ours was a living, breathing six-year-old girl with cystic fibrosis who came to our first full day of medical school with her mother and sat around a conference table telling us about what it was like to suffer from CF—but also, what it was like to live despite CF. I think meeting her on these terms, instead of in the hospital, helped set the tone for every encounter that followed. I might someday see her in the hospital on a pediatric rotation, but she would forever be a girl first and a patient second.

Not everyone uses God-language to describe this phenomenon. In most medical schools, this is called "humanism in medicine," but it amounts to the same thing. The language of advocates of humanism in medicine speak of dignity, of wholeness, of uniqueness—the same qualities that I am ascribing to the Divineness in each of us.

Healing People, Not Patients

Seeing the humanity in patients from the outset has meant remembering that they have the capacity for emotion: love, anger, sadness, worry, inspiration, and even amusement. My last patient encounter last night took twice as long as booked—because we couldn't stop making each other, and the med student, laugh. We had so much fun the woman invited my student for tea the next afternoon. You can't banter with a disease or an organ system like that—only with a human being.

A human gropes for the box of tissues in the exam room, wiping away tears that refuse to be wiped away, as they take in the crushing news of a cancer diagnosis. A human feels relief when they hear me tell them that they don't need to feel shame for the way that agoraphobia makes them act. Humanity looks like the proudly displayed photographs of a daughter graduating high school brought to show me at an appointment. Humanity is also the seat of traits like resilience and fragility, suspicion and trust, equanimity and intensity. It is the source of connections, both "supports" and "entanglements," that place the person in the context of a wider world. It is the source of free will—that intangible force that allows a person to decipher the genetic code they're programmed with, read the destiny written in their upbringing and environment, and say, "Not today it isn't! This is not all that I am!"

Dealing with souls is intense, like flying as close as you can to the sun. One of the greatest dilemmas I face every day is how close to fly before my wings melt. Can I handle one more drama of a broken, feuding family, or will that be the story that puts me over the edge, makes me crash and burn? My friend Jack once pointedly asked me, "If you deal with every patient on that level, don't you burn out eventually?"

Every six months in residency, we had one-on-one reviews with our program director. Burnout was frequently the main topic. We'd sit at his desk and go over the Maslach Burnout Index, a long questionnaire asking me how strongly I agree or disagree with such statements as, "I sometimes treat patients as though they were impersonal objects," and "sometimes, I don't really care what happens to the patients I take care of."

I heard Jack's question and thought back to those residency reviews, in an overheated office with a rain-streaked window that seemed a microcosm of the whole residency experience. I thought of how I fought like hell, despite the worst things residency could throw at me, for example, the pediatric ICU and the oncology ward and the remedial interns I had to supervise, in order to never voice the slightest agreement with those statements.

"Jack," I said, "not dealing with every patient that way is the *definition* of being burnt out. The fact that I can deal with souls and not just bodies every day is my reason to keep doing this."

I thought back to the summer of 2000. The world had not ended as feared the previous New Year's Eve. I had one last summer vacation on my hands, and I was using it to explore the intersection between my new career choice and the one I had discarded, by following chaplains around the hospital.

"I like stories," said the rabbi.

Rabbi Heimer spent his days listening to stories—stories from patients with unexplained paralytic illnesses, failed liver transplants, and end-stage heart failure. Like all rabbis, there was never just a story—every story had layers of meaning, the plain words and what they insinuated, the symbolism, and the deep dark secrets, piled on top of each other. He took me in to meet these fascinating people, to absorb the stories they told, and to show me how he helped them unpack the layers, spread them out on the table, and make sense of them.

Diana, a young, recently married woman, debilitated by a disease that didn't have a name yet, reminded me a lot of Assaf, deeply religious in every moment, always feeling God's presence. She told us how she had been raised in a Christian faith that taught her to never be afraid. They quoted a story common to both of our faiths, the first chapter of Joshua that ends, "Only be strong and of good courage." God expected her to be strong, she said, and fear was a sign of weakness and wavering. It was fine to be physically weak, because that was simply the nature of her disease, but her soul had to be strong.

"What if," said the rabbi, "you're confusing being afraid with losing your faith? What if God gave you permission to feel fear, as long as you continue to believe that God will help you *face* your fears?" He offered stories of his own, and a revisiting of the verse from Joshua. Courage wasn't the lack of fear, he said, it was determining to face things, *even though* we are afraid. As we left, she was pondering over this new angle—fear wasn't off limits, only despair. She could be afraid, and God would come hold her hand, even pick her up, and reassure her. She thought she could do this and still be a believer in her tradition.

Outside the room, he told me about his favorite story. "I love the Exodus story, about the Israelites coming out of Egypt." Egypt isn't just a place on the map, it's a frame of mind, a feeling of being stuck in a narrow place from which you can't extricate yourself. It's being parked in at the curb, with no way to find the driver of the other two cars. It's being pressed between two other bodies in a restless crowd, suffocating from heat and sweat and the scent of fear.

Illness, he explained, is like Egypt, a narrow place where people get stuck. They can't breathe, and they're stuck carrying around heavy tanks of oxygen that run out of gas (literally) halfway through an errand. They can't stand up straight from chronic back pain, ever since they fell six feet from a rickety stepladder at work, or out of a dead, rotting tree they climbed when they were 10 years old. They keep getting fired from promising jobs, because their ADHD prevents them from concentrating, or because their bipolar disorder makes them so irritable that they can't help getting into arguments with their coworkers. They're stuck drifting from one hourly, low-wage position to the next—or to nothing at all.

Healing People, Not Patients

Diana, he reasoned, was stuck with this mysterious weakness and debility, and compounding it by not letting herself experience the legitimate emotion of fear, which might have allowed her to release the terrible secret she was keeping to herself. She was afraid she might not be able to walk, or hold her kids, or do normal things, ever again.

The brilliance of the Exodus story is that there's a way *out* of the narrow place; someone comes along and hears you crying out and says, "This is not the way it's supposed to be." People are supposed to be well, not sick. People are supposed to feel secure, not scared, and there is a way to make that happen. In the story, God makes that happen. In the real world, it's up to us to walk in God's footsteps. Us—the chaplains and the doctors, the people whose job it was to heal the hurt and make the narrow place just wide enough for someone to wiggle out again. Letting Diana feel fear and not feel guilty about it was a way of allowing her not to feel hemmed in anymore.

I wish I could report back on the miraculous effect the encounter had on Diana, but with the way my summer was set up, I didn't get to talk with her again. I found this frustrating, until I sat down with a book the rabbi had given me, entitled, *To Walk in God's Ways*. Written by another rabbi who was *also* a hospital chaplain, it was a manual for performing the religious obligation of visiting the sick. The title was a reminder that this obligation exists because we believe that God visits the sick—starting with a house call God made to Abraham, after the patriarch had circumcised himself at age 99. If God can take a break from His Divine Schedule to visit the sick, the rest of us can clearly spare a few minutes.

My "take-home message" from that summer, then, was that if I wanted to be a nice Jewish doctor, I needed to be able to spare a few minutes. I needed to walk in God's ways by visiting with the sick. Not just rounding on them in the hurried style of most overworked hospital doctors, but really coming to see them, be with them, and hear their stories. I didn't even have to say anything "brilliant" (a real challenge for me—I love to listen, but I am pathologically unable to stop talking sometimes).

One of the stories in the book the rabbi gave me features a student who goes to visit his sick teacher and heals him simply by cleaning up the house and opening the windows, without even exchanging a word. I just needed to be there. I might never know what the effect of that presence was—but the person I shared it with would remember. If recognizing the Kiss of God in a patient means treating them as if we're standing before God directly, then recognizing it in ourselves means understanding that being human involves the capacity to do more than just mechanically meet our own needs. Humanity is the capacity to free people from dire straits; visit people in their sickbeds; clothe the naked; free captives; bury the dead; comfort mourners; and yes, heal the sick. We have the capacity to do acts of loving-kindness.

"Love" is a strange word to use in the context of a doctor-patient relationship; it seems to fly in the face of the detachment and professionalism that have been taught to aspiring doctors for centuries. But, a couple years ago, I came across a piece by

Jonathan Kole in the *Annals of Internal Medicine*. Kole didn't just *use* the word "Love," he advocated making it a fixed habit in the care of every patient:

> *"Our patient is a 19-year-old man new to the shelter, with a history of heroin use who presents with a small circular rash on his left forearm. He first noticed the …*
>
> *"Stop." Dr. G lifted his hand. "You missed something. You may not have been taught this yet, but I encourage a slight change in the typical presentation."*
>
> *Apprehensively, I waited.*
>
> *"Tell me why you love him." My mind raced, and Dr. G began to laugh. "No, not romantic love … instead, the deep respect, the caritas one might feel for all of humanity. Make that your second sentence."*
>
> *I paused, then tried it again. "My patient is a 19-year-old man with a rash. I love his passionate, personal artistry, his depiction of his struggles with homelessness serving as his reminder not to return to drugs. It is both inspiring and beautiful."*
>
> *Dr. G smiled widely. "Much better! Thank you."*
>
> *… Dr. G and his "slight modification" most molded me into the doctor I had always intended to be. Finding that second sentence has become essential to every new patient encounter.*
>
> *"What do I love most about this person?*
>
> *"Everyone carries a masterpiece in their pocket, a unique passion that they yearn to reveal. Have I found it?"*

I don't tell my patients I love them out loud, yet this brand of love pervades my day. What I love about human beings is that our divine spark means that we defy prediction and confound categorization. Bounce a billiard ball off the rail of the table at a certain angle, and you can tell exactly where it will end up. But, send a human being careening through the series of collisions that make up one life on earth, and there is no telling what may happen. It is this unpredictability, this uniqueness, this creativity, that I love, both because it is endlessly fascinating, and because it moves me.

One man may be driven from his home, chased out from beneath his vine and fig tree and stripped of the small empire he has built for himself, and spend the rest of his days with a tiny trickle of tears welling up from the corner of his eye without cease. A different woman from a different part of the globe may be savaged by an angry partner with words and fist, only to rise from the ashes and marshal every resource she can think of to save the next woman whose partner dares to try such things. One breaks my heart, the other strengthens it, but both touch it. Their lives are their masterpiece, their creations, and I have a front row seat to this drama.

Love, though, is something more than sitting in the front row. For it to really be love, we need to be on stage together. I could write a book composed entirely of the gut-wrenching stories of people I care for who have survived war, domestic abuse, and critical illness, but those are *their* stories. Saying I love them for their courage or for their tears is like saying, "I loved that show," as I exit the theater. To really mean my second sentence takes something beyond a theater review—being in the front row is not enough.

The day I met the woman who told me I was next to God, she greeted me in the way that all of my patients from her country do: by pressing her palms and fingers together in front of her face, leaning her head slightly forward, and saying *namaste*. "The God within me salutes the God within you." Love like Kole is talking about begins when my Divine spark can look into the mirror of her eyes and see *her* Divine spark. It is an empathetic love, founded on the visceral bond of feeling that we are cut from the same cloth, hewn from the same stone, carved from the same tree—even if, as my friend Pastor Rich Freeman likes to say, "Our tree is the same, but the bark is different."

That flash of recognition is powerful, because it propels me out of the front row seat and onto the stage. The landlord isn't just evicting someone else anymore—I feel like *I'm* being tossed out to the curb with all my belongings. Their problem becomes my problem, the solution my responsibility. The rage, the pain, the sadness, and the disbelief that emanate from the events in the story are emanating through me, not just swirling around me. I'm no longer the audience—I'm an actor. And once we are acting together in the same drama, reading the same script, we aren't just in conversation anymore—we are in covenant.

I'm on the front porch swing, writing during a thunderstorm, in the only dry spot in a downpour. Inside, my three children are asleep. When each of them was born, I held a warm, soft baby in my arms and made a promise that I would go to the ends of the earth to provide them with the only dry spot in any downpour—or else get soaked with them in the rain. Dry as I am at the moment, I have been drenched to the bone with them more times than I can count—and they still think I'm the best. That is covenant.

Covenant is mutual promises. Covenant is when someone else's problems are no longer merely of interest to you—they are now *your own* problems. It's what the great 20th century rabbi Aryeh Levine meant when he said to a doctor, "My wife's feet are hurting us." You feel another's pain, cry another's tears, and die a little death each time the letters "CTB" appear on a pager or text message next to the name of one of your patients.

When you're in covenant with someone you're caring for medically, your first inclination isn't to reach for the prescription pad or the stethoscope—it's to listen, to find out how they're doing, to visit with them in their illness. It's keeping faith with those who, figuratively, are sleeping in the dust, even if that dust is the dust of a career, a broken relationship, or a lost homeland. Whether they are a newborn child struggling to take her first breath, or a tired old insurance salesman waiting around to draw his last, it's promising them that you'll walk with them every step of the journey.

Creating a covenant like that between doctor and patient is a monumental challenge. It's a challenge, because every step of that journey requires action, decisions, care, and precision. Covenant means knowing how to walk the fine lines between doing right and wrong, too little and too much. It's a challenge because it may be easy to love a newborn baby and promise him the world, but much more complex and sometimes downright maddening, to love an older human being that walks and talks. And finally, it's a challenge because even when everyone has the best of intentions, building a covenantal relationship in the current healthcare system is about as easy as building a house on the Carolina coast and not having it destroyed by a hurricane.

As such, a hurricane is what modern medical practice feels like sometimes. Just when you have reached the point of committing to do whatever it takes to heal the person in front of you, a timer goes off. Their 15 minutes are up. It is someone else's turn—someone else whose needs will also be washed away 15 minutes from now. Getting drenched in the rain together, indeed.

Yet somehow it can happen. God and Noah somehow found it in themselves to trust each other and make a covenant to ensure the world would never again be destroyed, even though God had *just* destroyed it, and Noah's generation had done plenty to deserve being destroyed. Out of the rain, a rainbow. When we can overcome the warts and the flaws, many things are possible.

The red-and-gold clad women kept arriving, as though I was caught in a lost-in-translation version of Gryffindor House from the Harry Potter novels. Four or five times, a son in American attire, with an Indian college education, turned to thank me at the end and place me on that same pedestal. One woman even draped a silken scarf around my neck as a token of thanks. Four or five times I tripped over my tongue, unable to reply appropriately to this highest of praise, and said something silly or flat-out incomprehensible. Finally, one day, I was gifted with such an encounter at a time when no one was waiting for me in another room, and I had a moment to compose my thoughts.

"Doctor, you know, in our culture there is the God who is over everything, and next is the doctor, and we must do whatever the doctor says to be well. She was embarrassed when you offered to take her shoe off for her, because she must do this herself—as the doctor, this is beneath you."

"I've heard this before and am humbled and grateful to be your mother's doctor," I said. I was petrified; I have a tendency, as do many doctors, to defuse situations that are exceedingly serious with a lame joke, and I knew I would scuttle the relationship if

I did so here. My humor doesn't translate well into Nepali in the first place (I play a lot better in Spanish and Arabic), and I didn't want to demonstrate that my words lacked gravity. "But, I'm not next to God, or even close to God. Only that I believe that God made me, and you, and your mother, and there is some of God within each of us, like when you greet me saying *namaste.* I must treat your mother with the respect she deserves, and serve God by behaving as God would to care for her. God will never leave her, and I will never abandon her either. Whatever her journey must be, I will go with her."

Exhale. Pause. Translate.

She rose beaming, pressed her palms together in front of her face, inclined her head forward, and raised her eyes to mine. They were no longer distant or quizzical— they were twinkling. We had built a bridge across words, continents, and religions. Now we could begin to walk across it.

Get your shoes on—you're coming with us. I'll help you put them on.

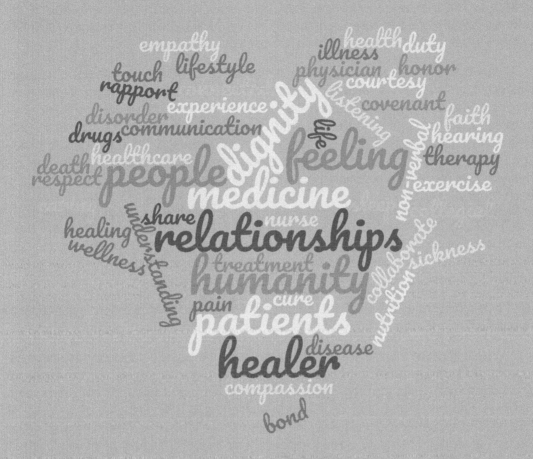

CHAPTER 2
Hearing, Listening,
Attending

There are six basic things all doctors need to know how to do. Ninety-five percent of my time in training was spent learning only two of them: clinical skills and medical knowledge. In the remaining five percent of our time, we needed to learn how the system worked, how to behave ethically, and how to learn from our mistakes (it's referred to as "practice-based learning). Oh, yeah, and how to communicate well, without which all five of the other skills are useless.

I was meeting with Kee May, a refugee from Burma whom I had known for almost five years. Normally, she came alone, but today, she had a young man, perhaps her son or perhaps a neighbor, standing at her side. All three of us were squeezed in-between the exam table and the door of the small exam room on our mobile medical unit, sort of a mash-up of a doctor's office and a Winnebago. From the outset, I knew something was off; her usual smiling face was tense, and she didn't laugh freely at herself or at me as we negotiated our little "lost in translation" misunderstandings of each other's cultures.

"I cannot remember anything anymore," she told me, "and it has been more than seven years." At 75 and change, she was old enough, especially having survived dictatorship and attempted genocide, to begin developing dementia. "I cannot do anything for myself."

I typed diligently, recording the young man's translations of her words as exactly as possible. "Tell me more."

"Well, it is more than seven years. I cannot take the bus, I get lost. My daughter has to cook for me. Sometimes, I forget to turn off the water in the sink or the bathtub." The young man waits to catch my eye when I look up and interjects his own words. "It's true. She has to have her daughter do everything, but her daughter doesn't speak English, so I bring her today instead. She is very worried, because it is more than seven years." I reply that I am grateful for him being here, as he has saved me having to shout through the static on my mobile phone to hear the translator I normally used.

I reviewed Kee May's other symptoms, the exhaustive list of questions that hopes to uncover the hidden cause of her memory loss. Yes, her stomach still hurts like it always did, like it had unfailingly for the last seven years, except when she remembered to fill the very effective prescription for Pepcid that relieved her reflux almost entirely. I suppose this issue might explain her failure to keep up on the meds. Otherwise, however, she was fine, except for this memory problem. No, she didn't have constipation, hair loss, cold intolerance (except what one would expect someone from the jungles of Southeast Asia to have after relocating to Pittsburgh) or any other symptoms of thyroid disease, and did not seem to have suffered a recent stroke. I knew her vitamin B12 levels were normal, so that couldn't be the cause for her dementia.

Throughout the questioning the woman's brow was ever-furrowed. Her expression didn't change when I had her move to the exam table, for what proved to be a long, tedious exam. I needed to do a detailed neurological exam, and each request

I made of this sweet woman was met with a look of bewilderment, and two or three failed attempts to complete the task correctly (despite excellent translation work by the earnest young neighbor). It wasn't that her impairments were so severe, she just couldn't understand what I was asking, and couldn't concentrate through all her worry. I choked down mounting frustration, repeatedly reminding myself that this was one of the gentlest people I knew, and I had no right to snap at her.

I finished the exam no closer to understanding what was wrong with her memory than when I started. Was she depressed? Was anxiety the cause of the memory issues—and perhaps of the stomach pain I had been treating all along? Was there other neurologic process going on? Or, had she really had a stroke, or developed early Alzheimer's dementia? Not knowing what to say at that moment, I held up my index finger to delay further questioning and dove into my online resources to review the causes of memory loss one more time. What was I missing?

At this point, it became clear that what I was missing was the entire point of the visit. "Doctor, she is forgetting everything. She is more than seven years in her English class and still does not know how to write her name." This seemed like a trivial concern to me, as I sat with my nose in lists of recommended lab tests for dementia. After all, she couldn't even remember how to cook anymore—why the worry over learning a second language, even if it was the language of the country she had landed in? She needed someone caring for her full time. Enough with English classes.

"That is concerning," I answered, with what I now realize was knee-jerk empathetic language, without really having understood. "We need to find out why this is happening—I'm going to start by checking the most important blood tests for conditions that can cause memory loss."

"Doctor, she cannot. She has lost her insurance because it is more than seven years."

I know what you are asking: what is it about seven years? The significance of that phrase was paramount to this whole discussion, yet until I had been hit over the head with it multiple times in the discussion, until it interfered with my agenda of "I must diagnose this patient and solve this medical mystery, because my doctor brain can't handle not knowing," I didn't stop to think what it might mean. You see, seven years is the maximum amount of time a new refugee can be in the system before they must either become a citizen or lose any and all government benefits—including the health insurance and disability payments on which Kee May was depending. Stripped of these, her mental health had deteriorated into a swirl of worry and sleepless nights spent praying to God to—well, to do something.

Or more accurately, to have me do something. She was praying to God, but aiming her prayer in my direction—except that until this point in the discussion I couldn't hear it.

Of course, I heard her words. I heard the interpreter re-fashion those words into ones that were recognizable to me. But, like in the old Simon and Garfunkel song "Sounds of Silence," I was hearing without listening.

People don't come to the doctor to engage in idle chatter. Especially when we have to be so stingy with our time, guarding a 15-minute appointment as jealously as we would Fort Knox. As such, the things our patients choose to tell us are almost always of critical importance. When Kee May repeated those words a dozen times in a visit, that emphasis should have been a signal to drop whatever I was pursuing and listen.

What's the difference, you may ask? I think of it this way: hearing is the basic biophysical act, like the cell phone commercials in which the guy wanders from place to place asking, "Can you hear me now?" When I'm washing dishes in the kitchen, while my youngest son is singing "Let It Go" at the top of his lungs behind me, and my two older children are fighting over who gets to eat the last brownie, and my wife attempts to tell me something from the second floor of the house, I actually cannot hear her.

But, when I'm concentrating on something, I can physically hear a sound in a quiet environment, yet it makes no impression at all, like background music during a conversation or the traffic that drove by the mobile unit while I was talking with Kee May that day. I heard it—but it didn't even enter my head. Listening involves doing something with the words we hear.

At the most basic level, listening is obedience, like when we tell our children to be good listeners. I say something, they hear it, and then they do what I said. Sometimes. I think it's safe to say that doctors often expect our patients to be good listeners—we give "orders," whether to take a medication or refrain from eating certain foods, and expect them to step on it. I think it's equally safe to say that most of us would balk at the idea that we should be "good listeners" in that way—whether our patients are demanding early release from the hospital, strong narcotics, antibiotics, or a second opinion, we bristle at being told what to do.

Obedient listening, however, doesn't work in a covenantal relationship, because it means someone is in charge, and someone is subservient. That's not a partnership—it's a hierarchy. Partners listen by giving weight to the words each other use. They assume that if something was worth saying, it's worth considering carefully what those words meant. We might be better off with the word "attending"—meaning paying attention. Not for nothing is the senior physician on a team called the attending. Not just because that person is in attendance, physically present, but because the attending is devoting attention to the patient's words.

I'm not hearing-impaired (yet). Kee May's question definitely reached my ears and my brain—but it didn't immediately touch my soul in the way that it needed to for Kee May to get the answer she needed. The answer was that I could help her get her citizenship by explaining to the Immigration Service that she couldn't remember anything.

Why is this type of listening such a challenge?

Ask any of my three kids or their best friends for rule number one, and they will all tell you the same thing: don't die. Medical school, residency, the entire healthcare

Healing People, Not Patients

system in the US is predicated on this same rule: don't die, or rather, don't let anyone die. The way to do that is by instantly recognizing all the possible things that could cause your patient to die and stopping them from happening, before it's too late. This is every bit as hard as it sounds.

My very first hospital attending was a brilliant medical oncologist who taught my small group of second-year students our history and physical exam course. In teaching us the art of the differential diagnosis (which is just what it sounds like—a list of all the different diagnoses that potentially explain the patient's symptoms), he encouraged us to begin with "the three most common and the three most deadly." No matter how unlikely, these were "can't miss diagnoses," the kind of diagnosis that, if not caught in time, could cost the patient his life—and the doctor her career. Heading that list more often than not was the dreaded MI: a myocardial infarction—a heart attack.

Close behind were cardiovascular diagnoses, like strokes and dissecting aneurysms, cancers of the ovaries and pancreas, ischemic bowel (the intestinal equivalent of a heart attack), and deadly, galloping infections, like meningitis, tuberculosis, and Ebola. Think of it fast enough, and you had a prayer of vanquishing death; fail to think of it, and you and the patient were done for.

Not all diagnoses end in death, of course, but there are other bad things that can happen to people as well, and these follow tight on the heels of the lethal diagnoses. Don't miss a diagnosis that could result in blindness, or paralysis, or permanent brain damage. Don't let someone end up deformed, or an amputee, or unable to eat, if you have any chance of stopping it.

As you might imagine, this makes doctors, especially newly-minted ones and doctors who are still training, pretty high-strung. Don't be the one to miss something really bad. Don't let anyone die. Don't screw up. Our communication has evolved toward this one goal—find the problem, fix the problem, keep the person alive. The medical world revolves around that sun, and it shines so brightly most of the time that it's impossible to see any other stars in our sky.

Patients don't live in our world—they live in their own worlds. Worlds where they have bills to pay, relationships to sustain and repair, responsibilities to discharge, and barriers to surmount just to keep going. I can suggest to someone that they need a stress test to see if they are in danger of having a heart attack, only to have them respond, "I'm in no condition to do a stress test now. I can barely get it together to do the really important stuff that I need to do just to keep going." No condition to do a stress test? "Wow—you really need a stress test," I think to myself, scratching my head. But, what must be going on in his world to make him too overwhelmed to find out whether he's about to have a fatal heart attack?

I'm not an emergency doctor, but every morning I read a half-dozen or so notes from the emergency departments where my patients typically go, and in almost every batch is a note about one of my patients who has presented for chest pain.

Each of my patients has a unique story, but these particular notes could have been cut-and-pasted verbatim from patient to patient. The patient says the words "chest pain," and it is as if they have cast a spell. A standard set of labs is drawn, including the troponin I, a sensitive test designed to "rule out" the possibility of having a heart attack. They are consigned to an overnight admission, and in the morning, they are subjected to a stress test, either on a treadmill or by way of a dose of medication. If they "rule out," which they almost always do, they go home. The "worst-case scenario" has been ruled out, so they must be fine.

As a participant in the ongoing sagas of these patients, I know that they are not fine. When I see them a few days later, they have a host of unanswered questions. "What's wrong with me?" they want to know. It is not enough to know that this one very bad thing is not wrong, because their chest still hurts and they still can't breathe properly. "Why do I have this pain? Why didn't they do anything in the emergency department?" I used to find that last question especially bewildering, since I was holding in my hand several pieces of paper that attested to a medical assault that had been carried out on my patient in that emergency room, until I realized that the meaning wasn't that they didn't do anything—it was that they didn't do anything to make me feel better.

When the man says, "I'm in no condition to do a stress test," it is out of a sense that there are actually bigger things going on in life than the specter of a heart attack. They may be other illnesses that are causing more distress, or financial worries, or broken interactions with family, but they are more important to him than 15 minutes on a treadmill that he knows ahead of time will not make him feel better.

The problem is, we're not very well equipped to listen to those bigger things. We start from chief complaints that fit pre-defined pathways, like chest pain, and follow a formula to do exactly what my first attending taught me to do—make a differential, rule out the deadliest actors, and fix the problem that remains.

Ironically, the formula developed in the mid-20th century, because doctors prior to that point were horribly haphazard in gathering information. Lawrence Weed is the doctor who developed the format of gathering and documenting information that almost all modern record-keeping uses. In a 2010 interview, Weed described the messy conditions under which physicians worked when he entered medicine in the late 1940s, a stark contrast to his controlled environment as a lab scientist. "A physician works in a chaotic system of keeping and organizing data," Weed explained, "and has no systematic review and correction of his daily work."

To combat this, Weed created a system of medical record-keeping that demanded organizing and titling the parts of the "database," keeping a numbered problem list, and describing the plans for the patient one problem at a time. He envisioned, and demanded from his trainees, a patient chart that was "the doctor's scientific notebook." Eventually, with the addition of computers to his toolkit, Weed was able to create comprehensive questionnaires for each "chief complaint" that listed all the simple questions that should be asked and basic physical exam maneuvers that should be completed for every patient with that complaint.

With the explosion in electronic medical records in the past decade, Weed's 50-year-old innovation has now reached the point where the record I use in the office is set up with templates for about 70 different chief complaints, and each template is organized according to Weed's logical system: onset, provoking or palliating factors, quality, region and radiation (location), severity, and timing. In each section, there are boxes to check yes or no for all of the commonly found answers to these questions, and perhaps room for one to two lines of free text.

I wasn't at work at my current office more than a few hours on my first day on the job, when my very first patient came in, a woman I had known previously from my residency who had multiple serious problems plaguing her. Bess and I knew each other well enough that we needed no small talk; I just sat down with her, fingers poised over the keyboard, and said, "So, what are we going to talk about today?"

"Well, my sugar was getting a little low this morning," she began, and my cursor sped over to the "diabetes" template. But, by the time it populated the screen, she had already changed course. "See I was drinking all this water to try to flush out the UTI I had over the weekend," she continued, and I hit escape to click the UTI template instead. "I've had three of them since the stroke over the summer that I'm sure Dr. Wolf told you about," and so, I opened the stroke template. Then, back to the sugar: "So, anyway, when my sugar was low today, I did what I always do, which was take a sip of Pepsi." Pepsi is caffeinated, and sugary, and both caffeine and dietary habits are on another "page" entirely called "lifestyle."

I chart while talking to my patients, because I find that like most people it helps me retain what we discussed; the longer my memories have to sit before being committed to writing, the less I recall. But, in this case, I couldn't even figure out what I was supposed to be writing down, much less where to write it. Weed recognized this problem as well. "Real problems always cross specialty boundaries," he observed in that same interview, and in my experience, starting from that very first encounter in my first real job, they also do not fit neatly into chief complaints.

It's not that Weed, or any of his successors who have trained me and my colleagues, wanted to leave out all but the first three words of the story. Weed's template includes a whole section usually entitled "social history," in which things like a person's profession, how much they smoke or drink, who they have intimate relations with, and where they live, are detailed. In encounters with children, it includes things like who the primary caregiver is, whether the child is safe from hazards like handguns (except in the state of Florida, where asking about this is actually illegal at present), unprotected swimming pools, riding a bicycle without a helmet, lead paint, and those nefarious objects collectively known as "choking hazards."

I teach social history to the physician assistant students with whom I work, and one of the things I point out early in my lecture is that we do a strange thing with social history—we bury it. We usually ask it after we've already finished the entire chief complaint and accompanying "history of present illness," so that we know everything about the patient's complaints before we know anything about the patient herself. This is the kind of relationship we might have with a bank teller—completely utilitarian, no personal detail at all. My wife once almost dragged me out of a bank shortly after we first moved to Pittsburgh, because she thought I was being too chatty about why we were opening a new account there.

In contrast, medicine's early giants, William Osler and his peers, filled volumes with witty quotations about how much more important it was to know the sick person than it was to recognize the specific sickness. Why, then, do we push off the social history so late in the interview—to the stage at which we are already glancing at the clock? We are creating a situation in which we might hear the answers to our questions, but we are strained to listen—or perhaps, we might decide that the social history is of secondary importance and dispense with it altogether.

Early in my practice, Kenny, a quiet man in his late thirties came to me limping. He was tall, thin, and dour, and knew exactly where the problem was. "I've got an abscess on my foot, doc, take a look." Sure enough, his left shoe was unlaced and loosened. As I slid it off and removed his sock, I revealed a discolored, egg-shaped mass surrounded by angry, red flesh and radiating heat.

"You need to go to the Emergency Department!" I exclaimed, not yet as well-equipped to control my emotions or mask my face as I am now.

"Can't—no insurance." We offer care on a sliding-fee scale, and in those days, before the Affordable Care Act, about 40 percent of our patients fell into the gap between being poor enough to qualify for Medicaid and well-off enough, or employed enough, to carry private insurance. This guy was one of them, and it dawned on me that either I was going to drain this abscess in the office myself, or he was going home to do it solo, with whatever he had handy.

Draining an abscess is fairly simple as surgical procedures go, but still time-consuming—gathering the supplies, laying everything out so the procedure moves forward in an assembly-line fashion, painting the patient that telltale yellow-brown color of povidone-iodine, injecting enough anesthesia to make it less painful (anesthesia doesn't penetrate an abscess cavity, so some amount of pain and pressure is inevitable), the actual incising, draining and packing, with enough caution to not make a huge mess, culture swabs, bandaging, cleanup, and finally prescribing antibiotics, checking on tetanus status, and arranging follow-up. I was looking at a solid 30 minutes and would already be well-behind by the time I saw the next person, so best hop to it.

There are few things so disgusting and yet so completely gratifying as draining a large abscess. The relief the patient feels when the pressure is released and all the infected matter is drained away is nearly immediate, and there is almost no risk involved, since, as a colleague once reminded me, "You can't infect pus." For a non-surgical type like me, it is one of the few times I really "get" the surgeons' motto, "A chance to cut is a chance to cure." And, indeed, this procedure was a success. By the time I was done, Kenny was able to slide his sock on over the fresh gauze bandage and tie his shoe normally for the first time in three days. He subsequently left my office with no visible limp.

I abruptly stopped patting myself on the back about three weeks later, when he returned for his follow-up. "Thanks for your help, doc. I feel a lot better, but now I need to talk to you about the real problem—I need help quitting heroin."

I was new, I was naïve, and I was in a hurry. I had skipped the social history to make time to drain the abscess, and it had never occurred to me looking at an abscess directly over the vein on the back of this man's foot that people don't just develop giant abscesses on their feet, unless they are actively instilling live bacteria under the skin—like Kenny did when he took a used needle and syringe from a friend and jammed it into the dorsal vein of his left foot. He knew exactly why the abscess was there—I hadn't bothered to ask.

I have since learned that little clinical pearl, that an abscess on the back of a hand or foot should make me suspect injection drug use, but I've also learned the much bigger lesson—skipping someone's social history is as large of an omission as not taking someone's temperature. While ultimately this man got into rehab and became clean, he could have been there weeks earlier, if I had heard and listened to what he needed to say. He could, indeed, have drained that abscess himself—I had seen it done by many of my uninsured patients, at least once with such poor results that the patient ended up in the hospital with infection spreading across her face toward the eye socket. He came to me as a veiled request for help, hoping that I would put together the clues and ask about his drug use, and ended up needing to ask me himself anyway.

Partially because of that experience, I now often do my interviews out of sequence. I lead with the social history and let everything else follow. Much of my practice consists of care for newly arrived refugees. Hearing their stories is far more crucial to me than learning about their illnesses—especially because the illness narrative almost always wells to the surface on its own, once we get going about life in the old country. Even with folks who are my socioeconomic peers, the small talk we make at the beginning of an annual physical ends up painting the big picture, be it frustration with their weight gain, inability to sleep soundly, or persistent pain that interrupts the work day at regular intervals.

It's not only the timing that's off with the social history, but the degree of detail we get that is often wanting. I spent a lot of time in residency working with folks interested in environmental health, and learned that 84 percent of doctors ask what profession someone is in when taking a social history, but only 16 percent ever learn anything about what the job actually entails, and less than 10 percent actually get sufficiently in depth to figure out whether there is any environmental risk involved. I don't have numbers, but if reading ER reports and consult notes are any indication, we don't do much better with the other portions of the social history either. When my patients who are Nepali-speaking are identified on their ER discharge paperwork as Filipino, we definitely have a problem taking social history.

Even the most exhaustive questioning in the interview, Weed's comprehensive Review of Systems, can sometimes come up short. During his early work teaching residents, Weed noticed that he could ask a pertinent question about a patient's illness, and the resident would have no idea, because it hadn't been asked—for example, not knowing whether a patient presenting with abdominal pain was sweaty, or pale, or had a rapid heartbeat, symptoms that might indicate serious infection, like appendicitis. He promoted the practice of systematically asking questions about every organ system, and lots of them, so that there was no excuse for not having asked.

When I was a third-year medical student with an obsessive streak, I made 5" x 8" index cards for each patient—they were pre-printed, so I could write microscopically small histories into the blanks, including medication lists, tick boxes for action items, and differential diagnoses. Under review of systems, I had pre-printed comprehensive lists of all the symptoms we typically asked about in each organ system, so I could go through the list in order, circle the "yes" answers and strike through the "no" responses.

Doing a review of systems with me was like trying to answer questions while standing up to your chest in pounding surf—you could open your mouth to answer, but all you would get for your troubles was a mouthful of salt-water. I never looked up, and never stopped to breathe. Furthermore, if I did get a positive reply, I came completely untracked. I then had to go back and do a whole separate "history of present illness" to figure out how to prioritize this new complaint of heartburn.

Every resident everywhere dreads the interviews in which every reply is a "yes." The reason for the dread is simple—just when we think we have figured out "the problem," the thing a patient has come to us to solve, more problems are added to the list, each of them a potential crisis in itself. Then, it's us who feel like we are drowning in the surf.

When someone identifies a problem in every single organ system, it's impossible to know where to begin. Some of my colleagues, acting in self-defense, have loaded their review of systems with trick questions. If someone agrees that, why yes, their teeth do itch, then they label the whole mess a "positive review of systems," and every complaint in it as psychosomatic. In other words, we are hearing the complaints—but not listening.

Yet, this "mess" is the beginning of a narrative, the story of the patient's illness from the patient's perspective, and can be understood by a clinician who is listening intently. The patient may not have even fully understood what story he was telling, until he has the chance to tell it to someone who is really listening. The trick isn't in booby-trapping the review of systems with questions that give us permission to ignore what we're hearing, but in creating space that actually allows us to listen.

Healing People, Not Patients

A favorite folktale of mine concerns an illiterate young boy who worked as a shepherd. His family had no money to send him to school, so he had not learned to read. On occasion, however, he would pass the schoolhouse and listen in on the lessons. As a result, even though he could not recognize the letters of the Hebrew alphabet, he knew their names and could recite them in order. On Rosh Hashanah, the new year, he went to synagogue and stood in the back. When everyone else began the silent prayer, he began to recite the letters loudly, over and over again, until the congregants began to silence him angrily. Finally, the rabbi was brought.

"Young man, why are you disturbing the others so? Don't you see it is time for silent prayers?"

The boy nodded. "Rabbi, I do not know the words of the prayers or the order of the service. I only know how to recite the alphabet. But God knows everything. I will give Him the letters and He can make them into whichever prayers He wishes to hear."

Even our most literate patients, but certainly those who are overwhelmed by the complexities of illness and health, do not always know what to tell us, what to ask us. They are providing the raw materials of the story, and we have to put it together, a task that requires time and patience.

About seven years ago, I arrived at one of the hospitals where I round, where I trained, before a delayed dawn on the second morning of daylight savings time. I rode the elevator that always smells vaguely like skunk to the fifth floor and found Mrs. M, who was tearful and worried, as always. In the narrow space between the curtain and the wall which delineated her half of the room (I told you there were still semi-private rooms in use) was the small bed containing this inordinately large woman. The rest of the room contained the tray table, which seems designed to trap both the patient and the bed in its vise-grip whenever we're not careful, two nightstands, the trash can, and a single chair, wedged all the way into the corner by the nightstand. There was no good way in, but I maneuvered my skinny self over there to sit down and hold Mrs. M's hand while we talked.

Clouds rose over the Fukushima nuclear reactor on one TV screen, and the loudly-narrated "crawl" of morning news headlines crept across the other, which wasn't even being watched—the other bed was empty. I worked my way out again and noted the clock reading 7:15, turned off the TVs, and squeezed back in again. The newly silent screens bracketed the clock, as Mrs. M overflowed with story, alternating between tears and resignation, as she described her narrow staircase, her determination to stay home, her confusion, and her fear. The hands kept moving.

I knew from my years in this hospital—any hospital—that this was not a common scene. Physicians didn't sit—they stooped, at best, or towered, at worst, over the bed as the patients lay supine staring up at the doctors' faces, like paintings on the ceiling. At this hour there was often a lot of yelling—waking up the slumbering patient, trying to overcome Mr. Jones' refusal to wear his hearing aids, or competing with the TVs that, like the one on the other side of Mrs. M's curtain, were left on for the viewing pleasure of no one. Chairs, if they could be found at all, were not in use, in keeping with the old adage, "The longer you stay, the longer you stay."

It was an adage we lived by in residency. If you stuck around to do an extra task, three more tasks would find you, while you were trying to complete the first. You could sign them out, but then your covering resident would get mad—and getting your sign-out "to do" list updated when there were new tasks to do actually took longer than just doing them. Make yourself scarce at the first opportunity, and no one could find you for more work. It protected our precious sleep and personal time, scarce enough to begin with without martyring ourselves over a lab result, a phone call to radiology, or the obsessive-compulsive need to re-check our order sheet for a fifth time to make sure none of the morning meds had been left off.

The problem with the adage was that it began to seep into our rounds. Time was always short, and never shorter than in the early morning with a full service and an 8 a.m. morning report, by which pre-rounds and notes needed to be done. Sit down at Mrs. M's (or Mr. F's) bedside at 6, and you would inevitably be late to conference at 8. The longer you stay, the longer you stay—and the evil eye was awaiting you, if you were late to conference, lumbering in messy and loud at 8:09 (or 8:35). Or worse, if you made it to conference on time, but not finished, only to have it discovered on rounds that your conversation with Mr. K had prevented you from seeing Messrs. L, M, N, O, and P.

So, we stopped sitting down. Many of us never sat at all, unless we were in conference. We ate standing up (bowl of cereal at the kitchen counter, before leaving home; sandwich in one hand, while reaching for the elevator door with the other; coffee, standing at the nurse's station), made phone calls standing up (and usually moving at the same time, once we got "pickle phones" to carry with us), and did sign-out standing up (in the hallway, hoping to finish by the time the elevator came, so we didn't have to wait for it to go to ground and come back again). And we rounded standing up, to avoid the vortex of the confessional, the convoluted story, the burning complaint awaiting us in the pre-dawn hours. The problem with rounding this way is that the conversation is less nourishing than the stand-up eating.

It turns out that I don't work any faster whether I sit or stand. Pre-rounding took me the same amount of time, no matter how I positioned myself. When standing, though, I have an acute awareness of the passage of time, whether it is because my back gets sore from hunching over the patient, or because my feet are tired from never sitting down. If I sit, I feel more relaxed, even if no more time goes by. Patients notice this. The yelling, the towering, the shifting weight, all convey our impatience to get on with it, the message that this person does not count.

The props we use for the conversation play as large a role in listening as does our body position. The residents' white coats usually have pockets overflowing with instruments, books, laminated cards with essential data and equations, and multiple communication devices. Even after graduating from that indentured servitude, physicians (except perhaps for psychiatrists) can be found carrying some minimum amount of instrumentation, whether on their person or at arms' length in the exam rooms: the ubiquitous stethoscope around the neck for most; the reflex hammers, monofilaments, and tuning forks used by neurologists; the x-ray equipment and viewing devices in the orthopedic office; or the otoscopes and laryngoscopes that are essential tools to the ear, nose, and throat physician.

Historically, and in many places still, there was a "chart," a manila folder overstuffed with barely legible handwritten notes from previous encounters, copies of EKGs and x-ray reports, medication and problem lists, logs of phone communications, and whatever other paperwork pertained to that particular patient. The chart naturally necessitated a pen, to make today's barely legible notes. The pen would also have been used to write on a prescription pad, pre-printed with the prescriber's name, license and phone number, and in this current, more suspicious era, usually some sort of secure background to ensure it could not be easily forged. Currently, of course, in most cases, there is a computer, whether a laptop, desktop, or tablet, serving simultaneously as pen, chart, and prescription pad—and as reference card, pocket guidebook, and phone call to consultants.

None of this, of course, counts the paraphernalia we keep outside the exam room: surgical instruments, needles for injections, medications, sophisticated imaging equipment, and other techniques and devices that form the impressive arsenal of modern medicine. As my partner likes to say, "When you have a hammer, everything looks like a nail." We tend to want to solve problems presented to us with the tools we have available and with which we feel comfortable—even if they are the wrong tools.

I spent too much of my time with Kee May fumbling around with my usual tools— computer, stethoscope, medicine, blood collection tubes—and not enough with my ears, heart, and brain. In trying to evaluate her "chief complaint" of memory loss, I lost something—I lost sight of the fact that her real chief complaint was, "I can't pass the citizenship exam, and I'm losing all my support structures." I forgot to listen.

I always sit when I can. I close my computer when it's clear that my reporting the information is interfering with the listening. On a couple of occasions, a new patient has taken so long to give his past medical history (45 minutes) that I have had to end the visit by postponing the physical exam to the follow-up, like a television "cliffhanger." I take care of other folks whose every visit fills double to triple the allotted time, so reliably that I am tempted to ask someone to "interrupt" me when the clock hits a certain time. I am pathologically incapable of being really rude to someone's face, and there are people I see who make me feel trapped in the room, because anything short of simply walking out on them will not be understood as a signal to stop talking.

Yet, what all of these "difficult," "talkative," "poor historian" patients have in common is unexplained distress, undiagnosed illness, or unheard grief. If someone, somewhere, had figured it out, they would not feel the need to talk so long, in such random order, with such desperation. Often, they end up referred for psychotherapy—appropriate in some cases, but frequently code for, "I think you're crazy and don't think any of what you're telling me is my problem." Our rigid structuring of the medical history, and the forced separation of mental illness, does not serve people with difficult stories well at all.

No physician worth their salt would shy away from performing hands-on duties like a surgery, a knee injection, or a cardiac catheterization just because it was "too hard," if it was something that physician had trained to do. Why, then, can a physician throw up their hands in despair and stop listening to an "impossible story?" As the man once said, "It's supposed to be hard! If it were easy, everyone would do it" (Jimmy Dugan played by Tom Hanks in the movie *A League of Their Own*).

What I learned from Kee May, as well as from countless others who have stretched the limits of time and overwhelmed my listening skills, is humility. I'm not going to figure this out immediately. I can't control the pace, timing, or content of this interview—because it's not about me. The 15 minutes you've been allotted may not be enough for you to tell your story. It's me who has to step back to accommodate you, not the other way around, because it's me making room for you that shows you that you're a worthwhile human being. And once I can make room like that, I may actually be able to hear you, listen to you, and attend to your needs.

empathy
lifestyle
touch
rapport
experience
disorder
communication
drugs
death
healthcare
respect
people
dignity
life
feeling
medicine
share
nurse
relationships
understanding
healing
wellness
treatment
humanity
pain
cure
patients
healer
disease
compassion
bond
health duty
illness
physician honor
courtesy
listening
covenant
faith
hearing
non-verbal
therapy
exercise
collaborate
nutrition
sickness

CHAPTER 3

I Had to Ask

My friend Martin has a cardinal rule: never ask a question to which you don't want to know the answer. It is a rule I routinely violate in the practice of medicine.

For example, no normal person wants to know the answer to a question like, "What color was the vomit?" or "How many pads do you soak through per day while menstruating?" No person with a shred of decency can ask a question like, "Has anyone ever physically, emotionally, or sexually abused you?" without internally begging God to let the answer be, "No, of course not."

Yet we ask both the first and the second type of question all the time, knowing that the answers will be vivid, horrifying, and devastating, as often as not. Uncomfortable questions, and their answers, are where the real story is. Learning how to ask them well is a high art form, as crucial to ethical, respectful communication as attentive listening.

On the other hand, if questioning is an art form, I occasionally feel like a kindergartener who has just spilled the finger-paints.

I sit opposite Lyle, a confused-looking man from two hours south of here. We smile benevolently at one another, and I begin.

"How can I help you today?"

Lyle tilts his head, as he concentrates intently on my words. Almost as if to signal that he is returning serve, his head tilts the other direction as he answers.

"You asked me to come in. I have an appointment to see the doctor."

"What would you like to discuss with me today," I offer, trying again.

"My health."

This. Is. Not. Going. Well.

Even saying hello to someone is a challenge sometimes, trying to be at once social and to set the agenda for the visit. Setting an agenda is crucial; getting it done in the first two minutes of the visit is actually a major contributor to the patient feeling satisfied and well-cared-for when the visit is over. In the aforementioned visit, Lyle does not seem to have an agenda at all; he's waiting for me to set it. When I make a second pass, he sets an agenda so broad that I could talk to him for a year and not cover all of it.

In principle, you might assume that setting the agenda with a broad, open-ended question is the best way to go, for example:

"What brings you in today?"

"How can I help you?"

"What would you like to discuss today?"

Lyle proves this approach doesn't always work so well. The first question could easily be answered, "The bus." The second, "I don't know—you're the doctor." And yes, Lyle would like to discuss, well, his health.

If open-ended questions yield answers that are so open-ended that all the meaning has fallen out, we might try a narrow, directed question, or even a non-question, such as:

"So how's your hernia today?"

"Thanks for coming back. Today, we're doing your six-week blood pressure check."

"I understand this is a pre-operative visit for your cataract surgery."

This approach is asking for trouble. Once, I was in the VA rheumatology clinic, seeing another patient like Lyle, who didn't really have any concerns of his own. I asked how his arthritis was doing. "Arthritis? I ain't got arthritis!"

"Well, why are you here today, in *rheumatology clinic*, then?" You know, the place where you go to see a doctor about *arthritis?*

"VA sent me a letter sayin' I got an appointment today, so here I am!" he grinned. "Speaking of which, when we gonna be finished? The van leaves for Clarksburg at 1:00."

Another encounter in a different clinic started out with, "How's your stomach pain doing?" "Oh, much better. It hasn't bothered me, since right after I saw you last. I feel fine." Ten seconds before the visit is to conclude, the patient with the stomach pain that was now gone casually asked me to feel his lymph node that turns out to be cancerous. We had spent 15 minutes reviewing a completely insignificant problem, which has in fact already resolved, because we didn't get to the real issue on the agenda.

In training, we call these "doorknob questions," because the patient doesn't ask them until the doctor's hand is reaching for the doorknob to leave the room. At this point, the doctor's brain has already left the room, having wrapped the visit into a tidy little package about whatever the trivial chief complaint was. Once the doorknob question is asked, everything has to start all over again.

However, the narrow approach occasionally yields fruit. "So I understand you wanted to speak about your back pain today." "Oh, no, honey, I been dealing with that for so long I don't even notice no more. No, today I need to ask you about my eyes— they've been turning yellow!" Offering one agenda, then leaving the patient space to decline that one and suggest another, has brought the real problem—jaundice— immediately to the foreground.

There's no one solution to the problem of setting an agenda. Every time I think I have it figured out, I show up at work the next day and have a visit start off like it did with Lyle. On the other hand, it's imperative to keep at the task of setting an agenda until one has been established to which both the patient and the doctor agree. If we want to listen attentively, we'd best be listening attentively to the parts that really matter. My partner often kicks off the discussion by saying, "What are we going to talk about today? You pick two things, I'll pick one." That way, she can grind her particular axe (usually weight loss), and the patient can stake a claim to the two things that are troubling *him* the most.

Whatever the question, it helps if it's a deep question, one that leads to a story, instead of a discrete answer. We all know that yes/no questions are "closed-ended." There's no room to expand on the answer. To get a story, I need to conduct an interrogation, asking an endless stream of questions. Eventually, it ceases to be a patient's story and becomes my story, one that I concoct in my head and then edit into something that only approaches the patient's real story, as I confirm or refute my hunches.

Seemingly "open-ended" questions, however, often reach a dead end pretty quickly, too. "When," "where," and "what" questions all have a single answer. Instead of telling me the whole story, I get one sentence fragments from a newspaper lead. Like the yes/no situation, I am back to interrogating almost immediately, trying to fill in details. Harvard emergency physician Joshua Kosowsky actually forces his students to do an exercise in which they are prohibited from asking any "when, where, and what" questions in a mock interview.

What replaces these questions, then? How am I supposed to get information?

"Tell me everything you can about the pain," I instructed Simon, the fit, athletic man who seemed incongruously distressed as we began our visit, ostensibly to discuss his leg pain.

"You really want to know about the pain?"

I nodded vigorously. "Of course, that's why I asked you to tell me. Help me to understand."

"I cannot work. I cannot do anything. It comes on so suddenly, and I think it may be my time to die." The mildly anxious demeanor and quiet tone he had used when he entered the exam room were gone, replaced by flowing tears and a palpable fear.

I worked backward from that bursting dam.

"Tell me about that fear of dying."

"My father died of a cancer. For many years before that, he complained of pain, and no one ever knew what the pain was, and then he died. I am afraid that now I have this cancer, and this pain is telling me that it's my time to die as well."

The temptation to rush in and reassure, to shake Simon by the shoulders and shout, "Don't you see there's no connection between the pain in your foot and your father's lung cancer?" was overwhelming at this point in the conversation. But, it would have broken the narrative, taken away the space I had made for him to tell his story.

Healing People, Not Patients

So, instead of shouting, I sat with Simon for a minute, absorbing the fear, before continuing. "You must see some frightening similarities between your symptoms and what happened to your father. Can you tell me about them?"

Simon gathered himself the best he could, still crying, and resumed the story. "Well, to begin with there's this pain. He always used to complain of sharp, stabbing pain, just like what I'm feeling in my leg right now, whenever …"

I noted the pause and encouraged him to finish. "Whenever?"

Simon looked confused. "Well, whenever—whenever he took a deep breath, actually. It wasn't in his leg at all. It was in his chest. Oh, Doctor, I feel so foolish."

"Don't, please. You were afraid and came for help. That was wise. Tell me what other thoughts you have about this pain."

"I don't know; I've been so afraid it was cancer. Could that still be true? Just cancer in a different part?"

"Tell me," isn't really a question, but it functions as one. It also functions as a signal that I'm listening, as much as sitting down at the foot of the bed or closing the computer or telling someone not to worry about the time on the clock.

"How" and "why" questions work as well as "tell me" for opening discussions. So does keying the conversation off of something obvious that I notice when I enter the room. "How did *that* happen, Joey?" said with a worried expression on my face is often enough to get the entire story, when I walk in the room and see a 10 year old with a black eye. "You look very tense today, Fatima. Why is that?" is as good or better as asking someone the reason for their visit.

Open-ended questions like these are supposed to give us a narrative. They bring to light a story the patient tells about their illness—or wellness, since not every patient perceives themselves as ill—that is the point of departure for everything we do. Listening to a patient's narrative is like reading a book or watching a film—and there's some pretty compelling stuff in these texts and films. Listening to the narrative in a doctor-patient encounter, though, is more like *studying* a novel together, digging deeper into it to find the truth and deepen our understanding of what's going on.

Often, however, the narrative leaves me more confused than enlightened. A wise teacher once told me, "Patients don't read textbooks." When doctors listen to a narrative, we're often trying to extract a subplot of a specific disease from the narrative of an illness—the difference being that a *disease* is a biological entity that behaves in the same way across the whole population of patients that have it, while an *illness* is an experience happening uniquely to one person, namely the individual telling the story. By telling me that patients don't read textbooks, he was reminding me that it wasn't the patient's job to "fit the picture" of acute appendicitis or Hashimoto thyroiditis—it was my job to find the clues to these diagnoses in what the patient was saying, and the only way to do so was to ask more questions.

I was convinced that Dmitri was having claudication—clogged arteries in his legs that were starving his feet of oxygen anytime he walked too far. When he walked more than three blocks or up a hill, he had to find a park bench, prop both feet up, and massage his calves. Anything further than 10 minutes from home was too far to walk anymore, and it was cramping his style.

"You can fix it, Doctor, right?"

Of course, I thought, except you don't seem to have any of the easily fixable problems that lead to this. Dmitri's cholesterol was normal (shocking for being Russian and over 60), he didn't smoke, and he wasn't obese. What's more, his feet both had bounding pulses both on the upper surface of the foot and at the ankle bone. He still had (considerable) hair growing on his toes and deep pink toenail beds with normal, healthy nails growing in them. He just didn't look like a guy with ratty arteries in his legs.

"Tell me again when this happens?" I said, figuring a second repetition might help.

"Walking, especially on a hill."

Hill—wait a minute.

"Dima, do your feet bother you if you lean forward for too long? Like leaning over a table?"

"Yeah, a little."

"Any trouble peeing?"

He inclined his head to one side. "Yeah, so? I am thinking this was my prostate, no?"

"And constipation?"

"What are you asking, Doctor?"

The hill was what clued me in. "Dima, I don't think you have claudication. I think you have spinal stenosis." Spinal stenosis, narrowing of the central canal of the bones of the spine, squeezes the nerves at the tail of the spinal cord so that the legs *feel* like there is claudication, even though the circulation is completely normal. It's not lack of oxygen, it's poor nerve function, and if it's bad enough, the nerves to the bladder and rectum can be affected as well.

Through some miracle I had him in the office of an excellent spine surgeon within the week, and the MRI images showed classic spinal stenosis. The next time I saw Dima after that, he was wearing an abdominal binder and a huge grin.

"Surgery three weeks ago. Already better, feel like I can climb stairs in my house like champion for first time in two years, thanks to you!"

I am almost never this lucky, just so we're clear. It's the rare story in which the only thing I have to do is dig out one clue and have the rest fall neatly into place, so neatly that a surgery fraught with uncertainty, like spinal decompression and fusion, which is what Dima had, goes off completely without a hitch and has such a dramatically positive result. Dima thinks I'm a genius; I know the truth, which is that I hit the medical lottery by having a patient who could clearly describe exactly what was wrong, and who happened to have a textbook presentation of a classic disease. These are the cases we all train for, where the only thing we need to do with the narrative is extract the plain meaning, then mine for a few hints at something we may have missed, and wind up with a diagnosis.

More often than not, hearing a patient's narrative is the beginning of a search for meaning that involves layers upon layers of interpretation, questioning, and wondering. What is significant, and what is trivial? What is to be understood at face value, and what is code, and what is symbolic of something completely outside the story? How much background am I missing? How many deep, dark secrets?

Take the simple word "fever," for example. I probably practiced for five years after residency before realizing that not everyone meant what I heard when they said the word, "fever." What I mean when I use that word is that someone has an elevated body temperature above 100 F. A fever isn't defined by the patient; it's defined by the thermometer. The only variation in the definition depends on in which orifice the thermometer was placed; a fever measured orally or under the arm ("axillary," in medical vocabulary) has a lower threshold than one measured rectally.

However, even I have different definitions, depending on which *patient* I'm assessing. In an older patient, I might call 99 F a fever (what my supervisor refers to as a "geriatric fever"). In a newborn, I would call a rectal temp of 100.4 F a fever and send the child to the emergency room; six months later I wouldn't raise an eyebrow until the temp hit 101.5 F, and even then, I might handle the problem in the office. When I ask the question, "Have you/your child had any fevers recently?" I am asking about numbers on a thermometer.

Numbers on a thermometer, however, are not what my patients are hearing much of the time. About three years ago, I began to realize how different the interpretations of the word fever were, and how completely I missed some of them by immediately responding, "That's not really a fever," if someone's child had a temp of 98 F on intake.

Some of the families I care for had lost children to infectious disease overseas. They weren't buying my "fever is our friend" speech, learned at the feet of one of the great pediatric teachers of our generation. Fever was a monster as hideous and fearsome as cancer to them, and demanded immediate action, emergency medical attention, and hospitalization, until the cause was identified and eradicated.

For others, especially the grandmothers who had never gone to school and were essentially innumerate (the numerical equivalent of illiterate), fever wasn't defined by the thermometer, because they couldn't read the thermometer. Fever was defined by the fingers, by the sensation of a flaming hot child in their arms, pouring sweat and turning pale before their eyes. Never mind the brilliant study showing that mothers are 99 percent accurate when they say their child does *not* have a fever, but only 22 percent accurate when they say the child *does* have one; again, numbers that didn't match their decades of experience.

For still others, fever, *"jora"* in Nepali, described how they felt. It wasn't a body temperature, it was a state of being—feeling warm all over, sweating, shaking, turning pale, and feeling weak and faint. One could experience *jora* right before fainting, or every night at a certain time, or when extremely worried. It wouldn't matter how many times I shoved a thermometer in your mouth to show you didn't have a fever—*jora* was something only you could tell me about, like pain or nausea. I couldn't measure your *jora*, your fever. Only you could do that.

Figuring this out is an example of something that is often called cultural competency. The more I hear the phrase used, the more I realize that we're deluding ourselves into thinking it is a goal that we can actually achieve.

Language and culture are not the same thing, but language makes a nice surrogate. In a sense, language is the vocabulary of a culture, especially if you consider language at the level of dialect. For example, New Yorkers and Texans both speak English, but their cultures are undeniably different. My wife just told me this morning about a man from Texas whose daughter turned to him, when she was served a grilled cheese sandwich, and said, "Daddy, what's this?" "Oh, that's like quesadillas, honey," he reassured her. Yet, no one would mistake this father and daughter as being from New York, once they opened their mouths; the accent and the vocabulary of their Texas dialect of American English gives them away.

Now, consider the fact that there are 6,909 languages in the world. In Europe, a continent with a couple dozen stable nation-states, there are 230 languages spoken, something like 8 to 10 times as many languages (and therefore cultures, at a minimum), as there are countries. In my office waiting room, we have more than 50 distinct languages and counting. We hear such rare languages as Matu Chin (Burma), Northern Kurmanji (Syrian Kurdistan), Aramaic (modern, spoken Aramaic, which sounds nothing like the Talmudic version I've studied, used in parts of Iraq), and Zaghawa (Sudan and Chad). By rare, I mean, "Not enough people in America speak this language for me to ever expect to get an interpreter on the phone."

Every cultural competency seminar I ever attended as a resident made me feel inadequate by the time I left. All of them were predicated on the idea that it was wronging the patient to not know their cultural needs and differences and tailor care to fit those needs exactly.

I attended a total of eight years of medical training and have been in practice for eight more and don't know anywhere near the full breadth of medicine or even my own discipline. How on earth am I supposed to be competent in nearly 7000 cultures, or even in the 90 or so I have seen in my own practice? It's an impossible task. More frustrating still was the fact that the people teaching these seminars worked for institutions that I knew firsthand had sent away patients of mine from scheduled tests because the hospital couldn't find a translator to figure out why the patient was there or to get proper consent. How was I supposed to work cross-cultural miracles, when they couldn't even complete a simple mammogram on the first try?

The seminars, it turns out, all had it wrong. My first boss, the director of the camp I worked at in college, used to gather us during orientation before the campers arrived and give the same speech every year.

"What color is an onion?" he fired off in his heavy Scottish accent that just begged for mimicry. After basketball, the official camp sport was imitating Barry's accent, often by repeating this speech.

"What color is an onion," he would repeat when no one answered. "Weinkle, what color's an onion, come on."

"Purple," I would volunteer. Other times he picked on another of my friends, who might answer, "yellow," "white," or "brown."

"The point is, the onion has layers—and it's different colors at different layers." We had to peel back the layers to see the whole picture. One of the things that had layers, Barry would then explain, was our knowledge. He had a room full of smart people— all were in college, most at Big Ten schools, and a few at Ivy League, crunchy liberal arts, or other prestigious institutions. He recognized that all of us thought we knew everything, and then pointed out that we didn't even know everything about a simple subject like the different colors of an onion.

"You all know what you know. For some of you, that's a lot of stuff. A few of you even know what you don't know," he explained. We could see the edge of our knowledge and recognize that there were areas we just didn't get, and readily admit that we didn't understand. "What most of you don't see is that there is a third category— things you don't even know that you don't know." That third category was knowledge so far outside our ken that we weren't even aware it existed, let alone did we know anything about it.

Cultural competency isn't about swelling the ranks of the knowledge we know with every imaginable fact about everyone from Albania to Zimbabwe. Cultural competency starts with an assumption that I don't know the whole story, that any person who is different than me in some way may have a priority or a reservation that I would not think of unless I ask. Asking blanket questions about, "Do you have any religious or cultural beliefs that may influence the way you approach medical care?" doesn't really help unravel that knot.

Just like doctors and camp counselors don't always know what we don't know, patients (and doctors!) often don't realize that a basic belief they hold is something that will affect their approach to medical care. The woman whose shoes I tried to put back on didn't realize that her taboo against letting a "higher ranking" person touch her shoes would ever even come up in the clinic, any more that I had any idea that me touching them would so mortify her.

In reality, I need to assume that even people whom I think *aren't* different from me probably are, and in ways that I don't realize until I start asking. The Jewish fast on Yom Kippur, the day of atonement, is one of the two most widely observed rituals in the religion (along with the Passover Seder), one of the last things to fall by the wayside among Jews who have assimilated into the secular world and as widely followed among liberal Jews as in Orthodox circles. On paper, all Jews who fast can be excused from fasting, if there is a medical reason why they should not.

Extrapolating from this, I know that when I encounter a Muslim patient during Ramadan or a Nepali Hindu who observes certain fasting rituals after the death of a relative or before a festival, I need to ask whether the same leniency exists for them. I know about religious fasts, but only in my own religion. From asking, knowing what I don't know, a kindly Iraqi gentleman I'm close with taught me that in some streams of Islam, a person may give a charitable donation instead of fasting, if his doctor tells him it is unsafe.

But, when I encounter people from my own religion, it's amazing how many times I trip over a rule that I think I know inside out. Some of my Jewish patients don't bother to ask me; if they feel a sniffle coming on, they will readily eat chicken soup throughout the entire fast. On the other end of the spectrum, my partner once spent Yom Kippur in our synagogue standing in the lobby all day, responding to pages about our elderly patients who had fainted during services, because they hadn't asked the doctor if they *could* fast, perhaps because they knew what the answer would be.

One friend recalls a night during his internship in Boston, where he took a call just after the fast had ended from one of the nearby synagogues, where an older man was lying on the floor, surrounded by off-duty physicians trying to decide whether to send him to the emergency room. My friend, having just broken the fast himself, asked, "Did he fast today?", only to have the patient bellow from where he lay, "You tell that young whippersnapper of a doctor that *not one drop of water has crossed my lips* since last night!"

In between, I take care of people who will, no questions asked, fast, if I say it's OK, and eat like it's a normal day, if I say it isn't. Others will question my reasoning and want to know if it's *imperative* to eat or just *recommended*. I often feel more like a lawyer than a doctor in these situations. Still others will ask me to dose their food and water intake, as though I were titrating cardiac medications in the ICU, in order to keep them healthy, while staying below strict guidelines established by their rabbis for "permissible" amounts of eating, while still being considered to be fasting. Clearly, this is not an all-or-nothing rule; there is an entire rainbow of shades of gray.

Getting at those different hues requires a question like, "How do you understand the rule about _____," or, "Something I'm doing seems to be making you uncomfortable. Can you tell me why?" It also requires active listening, like we talked about in the last chapter—picking up on the hesitation in the voice, the significance of the repeated questions ("Do you mean I *must* eat or that I *should* eat, or just that I *may* eat?"), and even the attention to giving non-verbal language of posture, facial expression, and activity. Miss these, and you will not even know that you don't know.

These beliefs don't always follow cultural or religious lines either. True cultural competency is really more about *human* competency—the recognition that we may all live in the same world, but that one world looks different to every single person that occupies it. It's the reason there's such a distinction as we made before between disease and illness.

Just like I will not always get the full story of a shoe taboo or a fasting loophole without knowing how to ask about it, I will not get to see the unique story of an illness unless I ask. Hence, my questions for Simon about the significance of his worry about cancer, and what the back story was that made him so worried that his pain, even pain in a totally different organ, was a sign of cancer. More generally, what's the importance and the impact of this disease process on the person who's sitting in front of me?

The disorder known as scoliosis is an easy one for a doctor to describe to a layperson the spine, instead of growing straight, curves into an S-shape during the rapid growth of adolescence, making it look on an x-ray like the skeleton of a snake in motion. It can tilt to the left or to the right, or wind front-to-back, upsetting the built-in balance of the different parts of the spine. It may present as lordosis, (concave to the back), in the neck and lower back, and kyphosis, (concave to the front), in the upper back.

Scoliosis is also an easy diagnosis to make without the aid of modern technology, much of the time. A teenager bends forward, arms extended and palms together like person poised to dive headfirst into a swimming pool, and reveals that one shoulder blade protrudes far more prominently than the other, or one hip is not level with the other, or the spinous processes do not make a single smooth arc down the center of the back. Standing straight again, I may see that she slouches asymmetrically to one side, the right shoulder much higher than the left, or that one knee is held bent to keep her legs even. In severe cases, scoliosis can require surgical correction to allow a teen to walk normally, make full use of her arms, or even breathe properly, if the curve is sharp enough to compromise the inflation of one of the lungs within the ribcage. Milder cases may require the teen to wear a brace, perform specialized exercises—or do nothing at all if the problem is minor enough.

Teen experiences of illness with scoliosis are well-documented. They include anger at having to wear a brace all the time, frustration with pain or physical limitation, embarrassment at not looking like their peers, avoidance of activities such as swimming, shirts-and-skins basketball, or using a shared locker room, and even humor in embracing the idea that "Hey, I look funny! Isn't that cool?" My experience, however, with caring for adults diagnosed with scoliosis has really opened my eyes to the spectrum of illness experiences with the "same" disease process.

Severe scoliosis is impressive when you see it. Norma, Karen, and Beatriz were all women with a marked enough curvature I could spot it from down the hall. Each had a hunch to her back, that from behind, made her look like she was in her 70s, stooped from aging, even though when she turned to face me it was clear that she was decades younger. In each case, the scoliosis was a source of disabling pain, enough to require steady dosing with narcotic pain medication and to prevent them from working gainfully since they were in their early 20s.

Norma would come to her appointments in tears, never sitting down. Sometimes, I couldn't even get her to speak, so deeply had she sunk into her pain. Periodically, she would wrench her back violently back and forth to quell the spasms of agony she felt. Other times, I witnessed her actually pound her hunched right shoulder and ribcage against the wall of the exam room; I guess on the theory that it would feel really good when it stopped.

Then, without explanation, Norma's mood would suddenly shift. In the middle of the interview, the tears would stop, and she would spontaneously hug me and thank me for all the help I had given her—all the while continuing to appear in just as much discomfort as she had been every other time I had seen her. She moved to another city after two years of this perplexing pattern, leaving me baffled as to what was keeping her so immersed in the intense pain drama she lived.

Karen was quite the opposite of Norma. She would shuffle in with great effort, propelling herself forward with her walker, and park herself in the exam chair. She unburdened herself of the tangled web of problems in which scoliosis was only the most visible. Karen had issues with her finances, her battles with other doctors' offices over her pain medications, her multiple other medical problems, her fraught relationships with her brother and her landlord, and her childhood friend who was her greatest advocate.

Yet, for all these other issues, the scoliosis stood out as the one which seemed almost to offend Karen. It was as if someone had afflicted her with it deliberately and maliciously, deforming and torturing her to no end and compelling her to engage in an increasingly chaotic pattern of behavior with us and those around her. She told convoluted stories about prescriptions, got in shouting matches with nurses and front desk staff, burst into prolonged, spontaneous crying jags in the midst of appointments, and finally simply disappeared from view.

Beatriz was at neither of these extremes. She came in like clockwork, and we would talk well past our allotted time every visit, running her list of medications and ailments top to bottom, punctuated by her dry wit, determination, and a healthy dose of "letting go and letting God." She made no secret of the fact that sometimes her pain relief reached her by back channels, but also made no bones about the fact that many days went by when she didn't bother with meds at all, because she couldn't be bothered and they didn't help much anyway. She knew she was short of breath because of her smoking, but also that no matter how diligently she tried to quit, her spine would never let her really fill up her lungs the way other people could. She never ceased needling me about my inability, at our first encounter, to hide my surprise at finding out she was under 50, not over 70, when she turned around. "Still think I'm an old lady, Dr. Weinkle?" she would say at the first opportunity in every encounter.

Despite their unique reactions, each of these women had a narrative in which the scoliosis played an essential role. So, it was baffling to me when I met Sunita, a younger woman from Nepal, one afternoon at her initial visit. She had immigrated three weeks earlier and, by law, had to have a doctor's visit within 30 days of arrival, which was truly the only reason she was seeing me. She had no complaints, no past traumas other than growing up abjectly poor in a refugee camp, was fully vaccinated, and wasn't pregnant. I was feeling rather useless, doing little more than going through the motions because the state of Pennsylvania said so, until we came to the physical exam.

"Sunita, is your back hurting you?" I asked casually, expecting this to be one of those off-the-cuff questions that makes me look like a genius, the kind where the patient says, "Why yes, doctor, how did you know?"

I was a little deflated, then, when she replied, "Not at all, why do you ask?"

"Well, I mean, the scoliosis."

"What's scoliosis," she asked, as casually as I had. She didn't have the mental baggage of Norma, Karen, and Beatriz, and she had surely never heard the word before.

"Your spine is crooked. Hasn't anyone ever told you that?" She had a clear curvature, and her right scapula protruded like a shark fin through the light blouse she wore.

"No. I don't have any problem with my spine." She said this in a tone that didn't mean, "No one ever told me about that," but rather, "You must be mistaken, or stupid— there's nothing wrong with my spine."

I didn't quite take the hint. "So, it doesn't hurt you at all?" I persisted.

"Not at all."

The practice of human-centered medicine is filled with missteps like this. I like to talk about the physical exam as being the practice of asking questions of the patient's body—asking the heart whether any of its valves are leaking, or the legs if there is a lesion in the brain that makes them walk funny. On occasion, the physical exam can reveal more about the patient than they realize, through techniques of distraction.

We do a tender-point survey, testing the areas that are often painful in fibromyalgia syndrome. In numerous instances, the patient's reaction to touch in those areas is more telling when we don't ask out loud, "Does that hurt?" They may complain of exquisite tenderness to touch over the tendons of the pectoral muscle, on the upper chest, and yet, when a stethoscope is placed to listen in exactly the same area and pressed firmly, there is no reaction at all. It isn't that the patient is faking, but rather that the mind and the body actually tell different pain stories. The body's reaction minimizes the pain, while the story the patient tells, describing their experience of the pain, makes the pain the main character.

There are all sorts of stories to be told by asking questions of the body, but we have to know enough to ask. There is a common trope in modern medicine that the physical exam is a neglected, maybe even dying art. I think it's no accident that the Stanford 25, a web-based curriculum designed to help reverse that trend, is being run by a physician best known for his story-telling, the author Abraham Verghese. While Stanford 25 doesn't express the problem in this way, Verghese knows full well that physical findings tell stories as well as words do.

My great aunt's gravelly voice (so striking that it earned her the nickname "Gruff" from the doorman in her building) told the story of her smoking. The scratches on the back of the 101-year-old woman I met in the ER a dozen years ago chronicled her life being cared for by her octogenarian son, who could barely get *himself* up the steps, let alone protect his mother from falling down them. Kenny's foot, in Chapter 2, foreshadowed our conversation about his heroin so profoundly it should have had a soundtrack of seventies music about drugs playing in the background—but I didn't know what I didn't know yet.

With Sunita, the story could have been told more fully by watching her move, reach for items in her bag, or sit quietly and comfortably. It was important to note that, unlike Norma or Karen, she seemed at peace, without repeatedly massaging herself, cracking her back, shifting positions constantly, or wincing. These parts of the exam would have attested to a woman blissfully unaware of a potentially life-altering deformity that for her was a non-issue, and would continue to be so, as long as her stubborn doctor didn't keep harping on it. A single finding doesn't make an exam, any more than a single sentence makes a story. We need to keep asking until all the blanks are filled in.

As a teacher of medical students, summer often finds me working with brand new third-year studentss who are good at knowing what they don't know—they assume that they don't know anything, so they ask everything. These students are as thorough as any medical professional will *ever* be in their career—and sadly, my colleagues and I usually harass them mercilessly for it.

"I was going to send out a search party for you."

"Oh, thank God, you're alive."

"She kept you hostage in there for a long time, didn't she?"

They are often conducting exhaustive physical exams on sometimes irritated, sometimes amused patients, without clearly knowing what they are looking for. Yet, sometimes they find gold, with the most notable example being the student who, while doing a very thorough eye exam during a routine follow-up exam, noticed my patient's eyes bulging and a "lid lag" where the entire outline of the iris could be seen without overlap from the eyelids. In doing so, she uncovered a classic sign of Graves' disease, a serious, but treatable condition, of overactive thyroid gland. Yet, we beat this thoroughness out of them with scorn, and by the time you get to my point in training, we aren't even bothering to ask serious questions of the body any longer—we're going through the motions.

My favorite physician-writers all have stories about occasions on which they went through the motions, and the patient called them on it—sometimes good-naturedly, and sometimes questioning their competence as physicians. Yet, this process of asking questions of the body can be just as dangerous to our relationships with patients when we are thorough as when we are not thorough enough.

Every pediatrician knows this. Somewhere around nine months of age, children develop a sense of what goes on in the doctor's office—and a grim determination not to allow it to happen to *them*. There are certain things that these children do not like having to do, for example, lying down for a belly exam, having a speculum inserted in their ear, and allowing a stethoscope to be placed on their chest wall. By 18 months, I can usually get a child to scream bloody murder just by walking in the room. If that doesn't work, saying hello or picking up an ophthalmoscope to look into their eyes *from 10 feet away* will do the trick.

Eventually, however, children outgrow this fear. In fact, most three- and four-year-olds have forgiven me for my earlier boldness. The real damage occurs later, because as doctors, we sometimes need to ask pretty personal, invasive questions of the body. In training, it was made pretty clear that doctors who didn't "ask the right questions" on every exam were both weak and incompetent. A common saying in residency programs is, "There are only two reasons not to do a rectal exam—you don't have a finger, or the patient doesn't have a rectum."

Around the same time that I was getting these messages, however, I read Atul Gawande's article "Naked," which lays out the two extremes of physical exam—extreme modesty, with both physical and personal barriers between patient and doctor, on the one hand, and grossly improper behavior and taking advantage of the patient's exposure on the other. We know patients often feel demoralized, exposed, and humiliated by being laid bare, or being systematically underdressed in hospital gowns. How much of this is absolutely vital to healing the patient and how much of it serves only to chip away at their humanity, the very thing that makes this relationship valuable?

Following through on expectations became a struggle for me, as each time I needed to do some sort of internal exam on a patient, I began weighing the demands of rounds and impatient mentors against the dignity of the patient I was asking to disrobe. In what way was the patient going to benefit from my probing?

The dilemma has only become more profound in my eight years in practice, since recommendations for yearly clinical breast exams, testicular exams, bimanual pelvic exams, and digital rectal exams have all been weakened or outright eliminated, as science has found that they are lousy screening tests for the things we were supposedly looking for (breast, testicular, uterine, ovarian, prostate, and rectal cancers). Why on earth, I think to myself every time one of these recommendations is taken off the books, did I subject people to this ritualized embarrassment to no real advantage?

On the other hand, there are just as many times when deferring to the embarrassment means a problem goes undiagnosed for six months, a year, five years, until it is too late. How else to explain the man I once saw with an incredibly painful penile ulcer that had been present for most of the calendar year? He had seen my female partner and mentioned casually only that he had some pain "*en mi cinturon* (at my waist)," which turns out to be a Mexican euphemism for "below the belt (also *cinturon*)," someplace he just couldn't bring himself to show a doctor with two X chromosomes. Months later, he finally secured an appointment with me, when he couldn't take the pain anymore. Women, too, are subject to this behavior, which explains the multiple colleagues I have with stories of patients presenting to them with cancerous breast masses eroding through the skin, because panic finally overcame the shame they felt at mentioning, much less exposing, their breasts to a doctor of either gender.

We walk the same tightrope with verbal questions that we do with physical examination. I mentioned earlier that we are in the business of asking questions to which no one else wants to know the answers. When we ask them well, we can effect some real healing. Not long ago, a patient came to me on pins and needles, telling me a convoluted story of a chance meeting with his ex-wife. He was making veiled references to things I couldn't understand and talking in circles, using hushed, conspiratorial tones, and acting as though he and I were plotting to overthrow the government.

"Stan," I finally interrupted him, "I'm not understanding your euphemisms. Maybe I'm stupid, but are you telling me you slept with your ex-wife?" Suddenly, the urinary pain and burning he was having didn't seem so mysterious.

The confidential space we build with patients, the trust we try to create, is supposed to facilitate conversations like this, where Stan can tell me about the complicated state of affairs in his personal life and begin to see the connection with his health. It's supposed to allow Kenny to be frank with me, so that when I *remember to* ask him about his IV drug use, he can level with me, without thinking that I'm going to turn him in to his probation officer. It made the space for Beatriz to be completely honest about the fact that when I stopped prescribing her pain medication years ago, she sometimes got Vicodin on the street, when she could be bothered to do so.

Asking the confidential questions, however, the ones adolescent physicians call the "HEADSS history (Home, Education, Activity, Drugs, Sex, Safety)," and which I refer to as the "sex, drugs, and rock 'n' roll" portion of the interview, can backfire, making the patient feel much *less* comfortable, or even downright disrespected.

It was Friday afternoon around 5:30, and I was digging in for a very long overnight call on the pediatric oncology ward. This was a hard rotation to begin with, but Friday afternoons were usually when complicated oncology patients became even more complicated, the time when implanted catheters malfunctioned, cell counts plummeted, fevers spiked, and unpleasant side effects from chemotherapy rose up all of a sudden. Either the children made it to clinic on time and got sent straight upstairs to the ward, or they missed the close of the office and came through the emergency room. Either way I was guaranteed to be surrounded by very sweet, but very sick, children and their extremely anxious parents.

One of those children was Samantha, an energetic, athletic 15-year-old girl from the suburbs, who seemed genuinely happy to see me. She had osteosarcoma, a form of bone cancer, and was actually pretty upbeat, since she was sure that the pain she was having in her leg was just a mechanical complication from hardware left from a prior surgery. We chatted casually about her symptoms, gradually working our way up to that morning, before her mother returned from the sandwich shop and sternly asked me to step outside.

"I don't know what you two were discussing in there, but please don't conduct any more discussions with my daughter without me being in the room."

I shifted uneasily—I hate conflict, and while I've gotten much better at handling it over the years, I did *not* have those skills back then, as a second-year resident. "Just finding out what brought Samantha back to the hospital this morning," I replied, truthfully.

"Well, let me tell you what happened last time with one of your colleagues, Dr. Jones, who will *not* be allowed near her this time or *any* time she is in the hospital from now on. He came in, threw me out of the room like I was the trash, and proceeded to interrogate my daughter about her personal life. Doctor, I promise you, she has *never* been with a boy, but this doctor asked her all kinds of questions about sex, and when she said no, he didn't believe her, said, 'Oh, come on, don't lie to me.' He had her in *tears!* I will not subject her to this humiliation again."

Needless to say, Samantha's mother followed me back into the room for the rest of the interview.

I would chalk this up to a naïve or protective parent, except for an experience I had two or three years prior, as a medical student in a private pediatric office in the suburbs. I had begun an interview with Brandon, a 14 year old boy who reminded me a lot of myself—skinny, bookish, more at ease with adults than with his peers. We were hitting it off pretty well, talking about school, his interests, and his minor health issues with allergies and occasional asthma, when the time came for me to ask the more salacious questions. I was being as professional as I knew how, keeping my tone neutral, non-judgmental, using normalizing language like, "A lot of kids your age are curious about …"

I happened to look up from the pad on which I was jotting answers down and saw Brandon hugging his knees on the exam table, blushing. I asked the next question on my list.

"No, and could we please stop talking about this? You're making me really uncomfortable."

If questions are about acknowledging what we don't know, both of these lines of questioning were based on a mistaken premise. My colleague, Dr. Jones, mistakenly assumed that he knew the answers to the questions he was asking Samantha, assumed that all teenagers were up to no good, and that with mom out of the room, he'd get the real answers. He didn't know if she really wasn't having sex, or if she was and was embarrassed enough that she wouldn't tell a stranger, even if he did promise to keep it a secret. Perhaps, she was telling the truth and had already been shamed by her more adventurous friends calling her a "prude."

In my case, I had assumed Brandon was *ready* to discuss sex. Instead, I found a teenager who was still as squeamish as most eight-year-olds when the subject came up. I forged ahead, tone-deaf to his needs, until the teenager had to finally tell the adult in the room to back off.

There's a lot of tone-deafness in the way we ask questions. I mentioned Lawrence Weed in the last chapter, because as he systematized the process of asking questions, he created a template that nearly all students of medicine since his time have learned to follow, and we follow it pretty slavishly. Fairly often, a hyper-competent, head-of-the-class medical student I am working with emerges from a room precisely 15 minutes after entering, inhales deeply, and, at my signal, breezes effortlessly through a meticulously organized, annotated history that perfectly follows the Chief Complaint—History of Present Illness—Other Active Problems—Past Medical History—Past Surgical History—Family History—Social History—Confidential Social History—Review of Systems—Vital Signs—Physical Exam—Laboratory and Imaging Data—Assessment—Plan pattern.

I can tell from the recitation that the interview went the same way: "Good afternoon sir, what brings you in? I see, thank you. When did it really start—morning or afternoon? OK, what part of your abdomen is it? Of course, do you drink alcohol? No, do you smoke? I see, you should really quit. How many sexual partners do you have? Really, that many? Any history of STD? I don't know, let me ask my attending if we can test for that (*a clear sign the student has never heard of this disease before, but will not admit to it*). Any blood in the stool, diarrhea, constipation, vomiting, chest pain, difficulty breathing, trouble peeing? No, not in public, that's not what I meant. Please lay down on the table. Say ah, cough, open your mouth, and take a deep breath. I meant breathe and then let it out. Don't hold it, OK? Now, I mean hold it, OK? I think that's everything. Very nice to meet you. We'll be back in a few minutes."

Weed, very early on, thought the process of interviewing could be largely computerized, something akin to the "decision-support" functions that a lot of medical records have today. When I hear a presentation like the aforementioned one, I feel like the interviewing has already been mechanized, without using an actual computer. What did this student offer to the patient that couldn't have been achieved by entering her responses into a diagnostic computer, like they do with my car at the Honda dealership? What's the purpose of even *having* a human doctor in that situation?

I'm enough of a Luddite to believe that there will always be a function to having human interactions—everywhere, but especially in medicine. Maybe it's my own arrogance in believing that what I do is special and can never be replaced by a machine. There is, however, something inherently worthwhile to that connection with another human being. We clearly value it even with customer service, the lift we get from "getting a live person on the phone" and then having that live person actually take enough of an interest to resolve our problem to our satisfaction. It makes us feel honored, valued—*human.*

How much more so, then, with our health, our very lives? Yet, when our human doctors behave like automatons, much of that feeling of honor is lost. When the pause between questions can be measured in nanoseconds, how much time can possibly be allowed to consider the patient's emotions, or register the importance of a particular word choice, or lock eyes and connect empathetically in a way that invites the patient to expound on how they are hurting? It takes a human to bring out the human in someone else.

There are times, however, when we are all too human. A struggling student named Carl emerges from the room, after perhaps 45 minutes, nervously clutching a piece of scratch paper covered in notes that will only serve to confuse him later. He begins the story in the middle, interrupts himself to say, "Sorry, I meant to say this is a 48-year-old," and continues to jump around the template, continually self-correcting to say, "Oh, wait, that's physical exam. Let me wait until I get there." Carl is either missing valuable information, or presenting it in such a way that it is impossible to relate to the thread of the story, despite the desperate attempts by the student to "stick to the script."

Carl's interview, I imagine, went more like this: "Tell me the story about how you got here. Oh, you're from Baltimore? Me too! Did you ever—oh wait, sorry, the medical history. Right (long silence from the student while the patient talks). Wait, I'm confused, when did the bleeding start? What did that look like? Oh wow, that sounds awful. Can we—oh my God I've been in here 40 minutes—hey let me get Dr. Weinkle, OK? Then, we'll pick up where we left off."

Speaking with Carl in the back room, I was acutely aware of the fumbling and sweating going on, as he attempted to put the pieces of Mrs. Powers' history together.

"She's 50, and her periods are always irregular, and there's this—oh wait, that's physical exam. I mean she presents today to establish care after leaving her halfway house. She's been sober for—wait how long ago did she …"

I held up a hand to gently interrupt Carl and explicitly ask him to just tell me the patient's story. I don't care if pieces of data are "out of order," as long as there is a coherent narrative that emerges at the end.. "Carl, what's troubling you? Is it too much information to synthesize?"

"No, Dr. Weinkle. It's just …"

"Something's concerning you. Tell me the story again—think of a drama, maybe a TV cop show, where they lead with the shocking moment. Then fill in the background, so I understand who this happened to, then bring it to a conclusion." I was thinking of a method I had learned in the pediatric ER, of beginning with my presumed diagnosis and then telling a story that leads the listener to that conclusion.

"OK—I mean, I don't know how to tell you these things. Dr. Yekes, my attending from last month, used to get very upset if we told things out of sequence. He told us we were giving sloppy presentations."

I smiled, "In your opinion, could it get much worse than what you did a minute ago? Life is sloppy, and so are the stories we tell about it."

Carl blushed, but laughed. "OK, here goes. Mrs. Powers is a 50-year-old woman about whom I am really worried, because on exam, I found a hard, irregular mass in her lower abdomen and pelvis that is probably 10 to 12 centimeters in each dimension. She's been having irregular menses and pretty significant dysmenorrhea for the last six months, but she figured it was menopause." Carl paused, sweat beading up on his forehead, visibly quivering. I was fully upright in my chair at this point. Carl's story had me feeling the onset of palpitations as well. But, I said nothing, other than to nod slightly to indicate that I wanted to hear more.

"What I really respect about her," Carl continued, "is that she found the strength to leave her abusive relationship and stop drinking three years ago. And because of that, I'm really worried that she may have endometrial cancer, and that's not #$% fair!"

It also wouldn't be fair to the reader to leave you without the knowledge that the ultrasound showed a large fibroid, a bloody, but benign, tumor which was successfully treated by clotting off its blood supply and letting it shrink harmlessly away. I'm still breathing a sigh of relief almost four years later.

Like so many other things, asking questions is a balance. We balance asking questions that are so closed-ended they leave no room for us to see the information we don't even suspect is there, and so open-ended that the patient doesn't know where to begin. We balance asking questions in such a rigidly organized fashion that a computer could have done it for us and asking them in such a haphazard fashion that we have only a patchwork of information instead of a clear picture. We try to ask sensitive questions, in a way that is respectful enough to create trust and invite openness, instead of provoking shame, embarrassment, and secretiveness. And sometimes, we balance our desire to know the patient deeply with the patient's readiness to share.

Pediatric HIV clinic, when I started training in the late 1990s, was a very strange place to be indeed. Many of the patients were infants whose entire existence took place under the sword of Damocles: as long as the tests came back negative, the sword stayed suspended. One positive test, and the sword began to fall, the young life decreed to end very prematurely in a single moment in the lab. When I returned to an adult HIV clinic in 2008, an attending remarked to me that the disease had changed so much that he was starting to do geriatric medicine for some of his original HIV+ patients. But, in those early days, fear of death undergirded every conversation.

Yet. Angeline was completely sanguine when I spoke to her. With her strapping baby Zion Joshua smiling and glowing on her lap, she was the picture of calm. We spoke for quite some time about what life was like in her native Zambia, where she was living now, and how she was caring for Zion. Angeline was HIV-positive. but felt fine, and Zion Joshua had been born after her diagnosis. The trip to the US was a utilitarian one. At six months pregnant, she picked up and flew here, knowing that if Zion was born in a US hospital, she could count on *something* being done to prevent the transmission of the virus during delivery. Now, 18 months later, she just had to hope it had worked. We wouldn't know with absolute certainty for six more months.

What was even less certain was Angeline's own future. Blessed with an unusually long symptom-free period, I asked, "What would happen when the disease finally began to take its toll on her?"

There was no profound statement, no wistful tears over a future in which Zion grew up an orphan, no expression of fear over her own impending death. I had opened a door for her; she walked right past it and off in a different direction. "I don't really think about that, to be honest with you. Just waiting for Dr. Steinberg to tell me Zi's results so we can go home," she smiled, and I knew we were done.

Doctors aren't the only ones in the world asking impertinent, uncomfortable questions, for sure. What's unique about us is our goal in the asking—the goal of healing.

My wife is a huge fan of the NPR program *Fresh Air*, hosted by Terry Gross. Nearly two decades ago, she was driving home from work, while Gross interviewed one of her most controversial subjects, Monica Lewinsky. Lewinsky was a couple years out from the mess with President Clinton and promoting her book, as well as a new line of handbags, and in no mood to talk about her past. Gross persisted, however, asking pointed, detailed questions, not so much about the salacious details that the tabloids had done to death, but about motivations, intentions, and implications, that got under Lewinsky's skin in a hurry. Unexpectedly, when Gross made her customary statement, "I'm interviewing former White House intern Monica Lewinsky, subject of the scandal that nearly ended Bill Clinton's presidency and author of the new book _____ (I can't recall the name); we'll be back after a short break," Lewinsky stormed out of the studio. When she returned to the air without a subject to fill the next 25 minutes, Gross opined, "She had to know I was going to ask those questions. I told my producers this was a bad idea, but they insisted. So I did what I do—I pushed until I got the answers I wanted."

Terry Gross is a journalist. Her goal is the truth, as messy as it might be, and her justification is that the people in a democracy have the right to know it. She's great at what she does. But, I'm not Terry Gross, or Mike Wallace, or any of the other great journalists in history who have made a mark by making people squirm. I'm not a prosecuting attorney who makes a living cross-examining people on the witness stand, and I am not a confessor who facelessly draws out the sins of the guilty and prescribes the formula for absolution. My goal is to make people better, and to keep them from getting sick. My objective is to ask questions that will help them figure out where the sickness is coming from and find their way out of it. My questions need to be carefully chosen to make the individual being interviewed agree to come back after a short break, not to storm off, before we've really uncovered the heart of the matter.

And if I succeed in all of that, I get rewarded by having to figure out what to say when I hear the answer I didn't want to know.

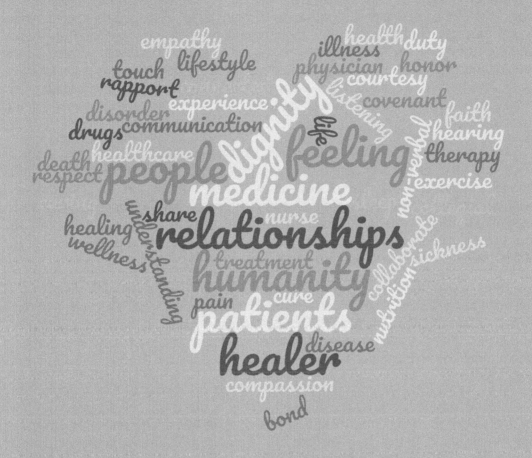

CHAPTER 4
Weighty Words

When people hang on your every word, every word becomes an opportunity to hang yourself with your own rope.

There are days when even saying "hello" to a patient gets me tongue-tied. The beginning of the encounter is supposed to be the time to tell long-absent patients how much they have been missed. It is the time to express to new patients how happy you are to meet them. It is also the time to welcome back those with whom you are already intimately familiar to resume a conversation, tackle a new problem together, or simply check in. It is the time for a warm appropriate greeting, and to introduce any extra personnel who are with you: the med student, the nurse or social worker, or the live translator.

For a handful of my long-standing patients, it is even the time for a hug, whether I'm ready for it or not. For some, the hug originates completely outside the clinical encounter; I have a number of patients who have known me since infancy—my infancy, not theirs. However, there are others who simply feel, whether due to attitude or gratitude, that a hug is in order. The number of times I've almost dropped my computer is more than made up for by the confused expressions on the faces of my straight-laced students who are also blindsided with a warm embrace.

Hugs are a tricky thing, and only work where there is a very clear mutual understanding—but the deep connection, mutual respect and affection that they express is exactly what the patient-doctor relationship needs. In an ideal world, every encounter with a provider would begin with the participants at least wanting to embrace one another, even if they don't actually do so.

Yet, even when the hug issue doesn't come up, saying "hello" appropriately can still become a moral issue. After eight years in practice, I still struggle with how to greet patients. My partner steadfastly calls all of her adult patients, even those significantly younger than her, "Mr." or "Ms." Conscious of a major power differential, especially in our practice where we serve an overwhelmingly low-socioeconomic status population, she goes out of her way to address people in the most dignified, formal way possible. Yet for me, this feels foreign. As much as I want to convey that respect I feel like addressing a patient by first name creates a feeling of warmth. "Mr. So-and-So" sounds like I'm working at the bank or valet parking the man's car; "Jim," on the other hand, sounds like someone I can have a heart-to-heart conversation with about—well, about his heart.

As noted in Chapter 3, I have other troubles getting out of the gate as well—setting agendas and getting to the heart of the matter. In a typical week, I see between 4 and 10 newly arrived refugees from other countries. Even though I have probably conducted this type of visit literally a thousand times, I can still open my mouth and have no idea how to explain to the patient, with the help of a phone interpreter, what they are here for and why I'm going to ask a seemingly endless series of invasive, personal, and possibly even irrelevant questions. "I'm the medical doctor, but first tell me about your experiences in the war 20 years ago." It baffles a lot of folks, based on their facial expressions.

If the worst that poorly chosen words could do was to create amused confusion, that would be one thing. They can do a lot worse. During my training, I stood helplessly as one of my attendings lashed out at a patient I'll call Marty, whom I had just presented.

"Do you mean to tell me you wasted my time coming to the emergency room at 10 o'clock on a Monday morning with this problem that your PCP could have treated—maybe even over the phone!?!" he screamed. I couldn't tell whose eyes were bulging more—the patient, who had just been diagnosed with Graves' disease, or this demonically possessed emergency doctor.

"I called the doctor's office," countered Marty, "and when I told the nurse what was going on, she told me to come right over here!" That had, in fact, been the very first thing he had told me in the interview, and I was certain I had shared this information with my seething attending

"This is a primary care problem! You don't have an emergency! Tell Dr. Smith he can start managing his own patients for a change." My attending stormed out and left me to bear the brunt of Marty's reaction.

"It sure felt like an emergency, what with the racing pulse, the drenching sweats, my hands shaking so badly I couldn't drink my coffee without spilling it, and the overall feeling of wanting to claw my own skin off!" Not to mention the bulging eyeballs, I thought. But now, all of that was eclipsed by a sinking feeling of worthlessness, even though Marty knew, rationally, that he ought to be furious. He looked at the prescription I had placed in hand, for a drug called propranolol, and I'm sure half-wondered whether this was some sort of placebo designed to get him to shut up and go home.

It was a public shaming. It was an experience scarring enough to make someone want to crawl under a rock and die—I wasn't even the target, and I felt like disappearing. And the most disturbing thing is that this was not an isolated incident—not isolated to this patient or this doctor or this hospital.

The old playground chant, "Sticks and stones may break my bones, but names will never harm me," turns out to be merely wishful thinking. The names we call people, and the words we speak to them, have immense power to do harm. It's not an exaggeration to say that a doctor makes a moral judgment every time they speak, so many are the ways in which we can hurt someone—or help someone—with our words.

Mrs. Street was one such patient, who came back to me positively livid after a run-in with a pain management physician.

"The pain doctor told me there was nothing wrong with me, and I was wasting her time. But, you believe me, don't you? Look at my arms! I can't lift anything. They shake. I drop things. How can she say there's nothing wrong with me? Look, believe me, I want to go back to work. Who can live on the $701 a month you get from Social Security. She told me I was probably working under the table—she should see my house! It takes me a week to get up the strength to wash a little bit of laundry, it hurts me so much. Why the hell am I like this, if there is nothing wrong with me?"

My colleagues are fond of saying that an illness has no "organic" basis, a more neutral-sounding way of saying that the illness is all in someone's head. My guess is that Mrs. Street's pain doctor said something like that to her, and who knows if his tone was sympathetic or harsh, or if his choice of words was careful or careless. I know this: when I tell my wife (a non-physician) about some of the things I see at work, she cringes in such a way that she has many times described to me as her ankles hurting. If she can feel actual pain in her ankles at someone else's suffering that she doesn't even know, I am sure Mrs. Street does not require an "organic basis" for her disorder to have pain severe enough to debilitate her.

Yet, we dismiss patients like Mrs. Street out of hand all the time, as if the only way to gather evidence of pain and suffering is hard science. The "data" that our patients' stories provide is discounted in its entirety, if physical exam, blood and urine specimens, and advanced imaging are unable to reveal a source for the pain. Even though their history is our entree into this patient's world, we treat history that does not correlate with some "objective" measure as inconsequential at best and deceitful at worse.

I'm reminded of a recent article about the possibility of an earthquake and tsunami hitting Seattle, in which science "discovered" a prior such disaster in 1700 or 1701, now known as the Cascadia earthquake. Local Native Americans had long been telling the story of the disappearance of the entire population of an island that clearly traced to that same time period. The author of the article laments, "It does not speak well of European-Americans that such stories counted as evidence for a proposition only after that proposition had been proved." In other words, dismissal and dismissiveness are a direct consequence of a failure to listen the way we discussed in Chapter 2.

Often, that failure to listen comes from a lack of humility, an unwavering belief that medical science has all the answers, and data volunteered from outside is useless— even data from other doctors. Even my patients have a pretty low opinion of the doctors in the refugee camps from where they came. I was having lunch with a couple of co-workers the other day who grew up in one of those camps. "The doctors in the camp would ask one question, touch just the part of the body that was hurting and write a prescription—always amoxicillin, paracetamol, or clotrimazole. That's it. Most of the people there died from misdiagnosis," one of them told me frankly.

With stories like this in mind, it's no wonder we might choose to ignore the data completely and start over. Yet those "incompetent physicians" have often helped me diagnose a difficult disease, taught me indirectly what meds work for sleep disorders and hypertension in this population, and what the expectations are when patients have stomach ulcers. Nevertheless, if the work of other physicians is discounted, imagine what happens to data we get from folk interpretations of disease, patients' own individual theories of illness, and social context that seems to just eat away at the available time in the interview.

I was asked by a mother I knew very well to explain the sudden onset of bedwetting in her seven-year-old, previously dry at night girl. Based on her urinalysis, she has "nothing wrong with her."

"So, why is she wetting the bed, all of a sudden, after not doing it for four years?"

The only instrument I have that can possibly diagnose this is a good question, something like, "What happened a week ago?"

"I can't think of anything. Everything's been completely normal, since we buried the cat." So much for "unimportant" details.

A different time I subjected a woman named Mrs. Needle to an exhaustive workup of her scary high blood pressure. I cannot name a single test in the cardiovascular arsenal I didn't do, yet according to the workup there was "nothing wrong with her," except her high blood pressure. Then one day in clinic I was beginning my physical exam, while still chatting with her. I applied the blood pressure cuff and inflated it, all the while discussing her life circumstances. The first reading I got was 160, but it hadn't been a clear reading. While still talking about her most recent argument with her husband, I re-inflated the cuff, and watched numbers creep up, up, and up: 160, then 190, then 220, almost as high as the day she first arrived, and I thought I'd need to admit her to the hospital. She blushed and laughed, as we both realized what had been driving the problem all along.

I joked at the beginning of the chapter that I have trouble even saying "hello" properly, but in all seriousness there are a lot of things that are really a challenge for us to say well. "You're fine" is one of those things; sometimes it is harder to tell someone they're OK, than it is to tell them they're really ill.

In medical training, we talk a lot about "ownership," that elusive quality that students and residents develop when they begin to think of the patients they are seeing as "their patients," rather than interesting people in whose care they are mostly observing the work of an attending. Patients, however, have ownership, too. At a certain point in an illness, they begin to own the diagnosis, the disability, and the sick role that goes along with that illness. They join advocacy groups, put themselves through tortuous training regimens to run 5k races to raise money, commune online with others who are similarly afflicted, and constrict their worlds to accommodate the limitations of their disease. Even at the milder end of the spectrum, people take ownership of the fact that there is no way they can make it to work today, or that there is no chance that they will get better, unless you do something.

When we question, reverse, or "rule-out" a long-held diagnosis, we are taking away that ownership. This is not necessarily a bad thing. My friend Peter runs a clinic for adults with Trisomy 21 (Down Syndrome), and he jokes that he specializes in curing dementia. It is known that Down Syndrome causes earlier-than-normal onset of Alzheimer-type dementia, which for individuals with Trisomy 21 who survive to adulthood is the "final common pathway" toward death, usually between ages 55 and 75. However, it is also true that Down Syndrome has a high incidence of pretty severe under-activity of the thyroid gland—severe enough to make someone appear to be actively dementing. When family members bring their affected loved ones to see Peter, they are often convinced that the dementia process has begun—until Peter diagnoses and treats the thyroid deficiency, and "cures" the dementia.

I have "cured" at least one case of lupus, one case of ALS, and a few cases of rheumatoid arthritis by challenging the diagnosis and turning out to be correct. I have also "cured" one patient of leukemia by referring him to a hematologist, only to find out that the pinpoint red dots caused by malfunctioning platelets were actually due to a severe vitamin deficiency and not to cancer. Each case, especially the last one, of course, was met with relief. Not all patients, however, surrender ownership of their diagnoses so easily.

"You're fine," or more specifically, "you don't have Crohn's disease/rheumatoid arthritis/a thyroid problem," can actually take away hope. If it's not that thing that I was convinced I had, what's wrong with me? Why can't I get out of bed in the morning? Why don't my clothes fit? And if you're so smart, how else do you explain the pain/vomiting/diarrhea/itching? Do you think I'm faking? Do you think I'm crazy?

I spend a lot of time with people with complicated, hard-to-prove diagnoses that lack a single definitive test. To a person, they tell me, "It took me years to finally get diagnosed with this. No one believed me that I had this disease," whether the illness in question is mitochondrial disease, malalignment of a part of the body that does not usually mal-align, or mast-cell destabilization disorder.

Many of these patients have become activists around their diagnosis, joined online communities, and advocated to "spread the word" about their sickness. The diagnosis, a specific name for their suffering, has given them an explanation for their troubles. Sometimes, I have to admit, it may provide an excuse for why they can't meet obligations, or a card to play for sympathy. Most of the time, however, it simply helps them make sense of why their lives are the way they are. If I question the diagnosis, it's as if I am trying to destroy the order of their universe.

The last 10 years of being in practice have been a struggle to find the right way to say, "You're fine," or rather, to stop saying that and replace it with something more exact. "You do not have a fatal or terminal illness, or a disease that will cause permanent disability. But, you do seem to have a lot of pain and unpleasant symptoms. Those problems are really frustrating you and limiting your daily activity, and making it hard for you to support your family." These people are not fine. They don't need to hear that they are fine, or that their heart, lungs or kidneys are fine (as often happens in a specialty visit—"Well it's not the heart. Go see your PCP."). And they definitely don't need to hear, "It's all in your head."

Except that they do. They need to hear that we do believe in the mind-body axis, that the brain is an organ of the body, and it can do screwy things to the rest of the body when it's under stress, and that this can cause a level of disability nearly equal to what would happen if the disease they thought was there were actually there. They need to hear that we aren't omniscient, that we own the uncertainty of our diagnosis, that we own our responsibility to stick by them until we figure it out and that we are genuinely sorry they feel this way, even though we didn't cause the problem.

In reality, some people are fine, and they need to hear it. They need to hear, "I'm so glad to tell you that you don't have pneumonia, and your lungs are clear. You're not wheezing, and this is a cold. There are no guarantees, but I would expect you to be better within five to seven days. And yes, you are fine to go to work. And Johnny doesn't have strep throat or pneumonia either—he's fine to go to school." The opposite of dismissal is reassurance. When we say, "you're fine," we could be doing either of these things. What we say after "you're fine" is what makes all the difference.

It's easy to falter when trying to walk the "you're fine" line. It's easy to perpetuate a sense of disability and learned helplessness in someone by over-validating their concerns, even when legitimate. I spent years as a camp counselor when I was an undergraduate (and am now one of the camp doctors at the same camp). Every summer there were a few campers who arrived at camp armed to the teeth with medications for every conceivable ailment, and letters from their parents issuing detailed cautions to the staff to watch for various behaviors, odd symptoms, and severe reactions. Every summer at least a few of those kids absented themselves from the best activities, or brought camp to a screeching halt with much ado about nothing. At the same time, at least a few of the others put on a good humor about their weird disease, maybe even adopted a nickname based on it, set aside the sick role and skipped med call more often than not, and ended up having the summer of their lives, without ever getting really sick.

Words, especially a doctor's words, can have a lot to do with which path someone follows. "I know how sick you feel, and it may seem like going swimming tomorrow is the worst thing you could do. But, I know how much fun it's going to be, and it won't actually make you any sicker to participate, so I'm giving you permission to go, and I think you should try," can lead to a very different day than, "Oh, you're right, you probably won't want to swim tomorrow; you're really not going to feel up to it, and I don't want you to overdo it. You can't play games with your health."

Both approaches are supportive, both are validating the child's feelings, but the first approach includes a, "Nevertheless ... "instead of accepting everything at face value. Treating a person with the respect and dignity we discussed in Chapter 1 doesn't mean we can't disagree with them or even challenge them—but disagreement doesn't mean argument, and challenge doesn't mean disrespect, unless we go about it in a confrontational way, like Marty's doctor did.

Part of me wishes Marty had the good fortune to see my teacher Peter Antevy in the ER instead, except that Peter is a pediatric ER doc whom I trained under in residency. Peter is well aware that the bulk of pediatric emergency patients "don't need to be there," since they have non-life-threatening problems that could easily have waited until morning, or Monday, or gone to Urgent Care, or maybe not have been seen at all. Yet for all the colds, mild diarrhea, ear infections, and "fevers" that weren't really fevers, Peter had an answer. "The first thing I say to every family," he told me one evening between patients, "once I've heard the story and examined the child and am ready to give my diagnosis, is, 'I'm so glad you came in.'"

Peter recognized that there was always a story behind why the child was there "unnecessarily": a nervous first time parent, a family with no insurance, a child screaming "unnecessarily" through the night with a trivial illness that finally sent the exasperated family to the ER. "I'm so glad you came in" validated that story, let them know he understood that there must be a reason they would choose to spend precious time in an emergency department with their child, and also gave value to whatever advice he was able to provide in the next sentence.

Peter's approach helps us deal with the category that many doctors find most frustrating, the so-called "worried well." It is a helpful reminder of the narrative that underlies every patient encounter. Even more important, if we can learn to validate the concerns of the worried well compassionately, then when we are confronted with more severely ill patients, we should be able to rise to the task of validating their concerns more easily.

I like to imagine Peter might have handled the situation with Marty much differently:

"It sounds like your PCP is really worried about you—that racing heartbeat can be really scary, and it doesn't sound like you can get much work done when your hands are shaking like that."

Marty acknowledged he had actually called off today prior to calling the PCP, since he could barely button his shirt—and once he did, he had perspired right through it in about 10 minutes.

"I'm glad you came in, then. Now, I can tell you confidently this is part of the thyroid problem your PCP diagnosed you with a few weeks ago—it's called thyrotoxicosis. We know this happens pretty often in your disease. Did he tell you about this?"

Sheepishly, Marty realized he had been warned this might happen, but forgot—and didn't tell the nurse in the office when he called. He began to apologize, but the doctor held up her hand to stop him.

"Do you think I expect you to think clearly feeling like that? Don't worry. Panic is part of the problem in this condition, so I'm not surprised you assumed you're having a heart attack—which, as I was saying, I can now tell you isn't the case."

Healing People, Not Patients

Marty felt a flood of relief cascade over him—or so he thought; it might just have been another gush of sweat. But, he definitely felt better knowing this was all part of a disease he already knew he had.

"Listen, next time this happens there's no need to come in. Just tell your doctor's triage nurse the whole story, including the advice I'm giving you know, and they can take it from there. But, if it's worse, or new symptoms come up, or it's night or the weekend, you can feel free to come back. Meantime, take this prescription. It's for a medicine called propranolol that will stop the symptoms—the sweating, the shaking, and the racing heartbeat especially. Eventually that anti-thyroid medication Dr. Smith gave you will get the problem under control for the long term, but that could be another month or two, so you'll need this in the meantime."

"Thanks, doc. I feel a lot better now."

"Good. Thanks for coming in."

This way Marty feels validated, justified for having sought the attention he did but at the same time we have successfully challenged the idea that he "needs to be in the ER," since the problem is known and the solution can be administered in pill form. He will likely stay home from the ER the next time because he feels safe to do so, thanks to the reassurance he was given, instead of due to the insulting treatment he received on his initial visit. He still has the sick role, but it has been ratcheted down a few notches by careful attention, accurate education, and respectful language.

Sometimes, we do harm with our words in exactly the opposite way, by taking a healthy person and through our words convince them that they are, in fact, quite ill. Dartmouth professor and internist Gilbert Welch calls this, "the paradox of promoting health by encouraging policies that lead more people to view themselves as sick." A couple years ago a man came into my office for a visit, and after my exam, he seemed to be in fantastic shape—and I told him so.

"I don't know how you can be saying there's nothing wrong with my heart," he protested. "The doctor in Chicago told me I needed cholesterol meds, blood pressure meds, and diabetes meds, or I'd be dead of a heart attack by my 45th birthday!"

This poor man was taking more medications than he had digits on his hand, and hadn't even reached his forties. I countered that this non-smoker, who worked six days a week as a bicycle messenger and ate a vegan diet, was far more likely to donate a perfectly preserved heart for transplant if he didn't start wearing his bike helmet, than to ever have a heart attack. He was unmoved. The fear of a heart attack had him. "So, you won't do my stress test? This place is such a backwater!"

Fear will get people to buy more than car insurance or an incumbent president, however. In the medical world, people will buy into treatments they may not need, and that may be harming them, out of fear of the possible consequences of not doing what is suggested.

Some colleague of mine in Chicago, whom I have never met and will never meet, has scared this incredibly fit young man into believing that he is on a collision course with sudden cardiac death (instead of the far more likely scenario of a collision with a CTA bus). He now takes five different medications in order to ward off that looming catastrophe, at great personal cost (he has no insurance), and at some physical cost as well. His stomach is upset from his metformin. His muscles ache from the statins, which make work excruciating. He has a cough from the ACE inhibitor. He makes constant trips to the restroom from the diuretic. It takes an agonizingly long time for him to stop bleeding from his road rash thanks to the aspirin. Oh, and the fish burps from the fish oil, which he hates taking even more, because it's an animal product.

Yet, when I finally obtain records from the prior physician, I find a normal EKG, cholesterol, blood sugar, and blood pressure. I also find a man completely changed from the description he gave me of himself prior to seeing the other doctor—someone who has gone from robust, happy, and determined, to tentative, edgy, and fearful.

It's true that, sometimes, fear of developing a disease is a powerful motivator for good, such as the patient who looks at his family tree, sees it covered in the dead leaves of premature heart disease, and resolves to take up rowing and give up doughnuts. On occasion, pre-disease does involve real risk of worse overt disease down the road, and can be a golden opportunity to intervene with lifestyle changes at a point where they will actually prevent the full-blown disease from happening. The dilemma, then, is how to convey that message without creating a degree of fear that prevents people from being able to live. I once had a bright 14-year-old patient look me in the eye, when I asked him if he drinks, and say, "You've met my dad and seen what alcohol did to him. I'm way too afraid that could happen to me to even touch alcohol." Sometimes, fear is also the needed element to keep people safe in an epidemic, natural disaster, or other hazard, where our natural human urges would otherwise make us sitting ducks.

Unfortunately, fear doesn't even work that well in many situations, as I've learned against my better judgment. The patient in Chapter 3 who caught me with my hand already on the doorknob and asked me about his enlarged lymph node had a non-refundable trip to Wisconsin planned for the following Monday to visit friends and family that he hadn't seen since moving away, and was not going to miss it.

Not knowing what he had, I imagined the worst, the case of Burkitt's lymphoma I had seen eat away at a young boy's jaw in a matter of days. "This is probably lymphoma, and it could be an aggressive one," I implored him. "If you leave on this trip before you know what it is, you may be dead before you come back." He was unmoved. I later learned why: He was as afraid as I was, but his fear had another dimension to it. He knew that once he started treatment, he'd be trapped. If he was dying, he wanted the trip to Wisconsin to happen while he was healthy, so he could enjoy the final visit with these relatives in peace. So, I waited in fear the entire time he was gone, hoping to hear his voice once again. As he approaches three years survival, I prepare to eat my words with a slice of humble pie for dessert.

Fear is also of limited use as a long-term motivator. A recovering alcoholic once told me, "Fear kept me sober for about two weeks. After that, it falls apart. In the end, sobriety wasn't about not drinking; it was about enjoying life without alcohol. Fear wasn't enough." People trying to achieve behavior change don't hang on to that fear of an early death or disability for very long when faced with a bottle, a cigarette, a needle, or a Big Mac.

Yet, sometimes real, irreversible harm often comes during the brief window when fear is the primary motivator. I remember a lecturer when I was a second-year medical student who described the case of a woman sent for a "routine stress test" for "thoroughness sake," because she was overweight, or had high blood pressure, or slightly abnormal cholesterol. She had a not-entirely-normal outcome. The obvious next step—catheterization, and fast; after all, we are trying to prevent a heart attack.

A cascade of testing was unleashed. The problem is that during the catheterization, this woman suffered a stroke—a piece of plaque from her aorta flicked off into her carotid artery and landed in her brain. She hadn't really needed a catheterization in the first place; now, she was disabled.

Furthermore, this woman's story isn't unique, nor is it limited to fear of heart attacks. The "fear factor" comes into play in cancer screening all the time, even as evidence accumulates that there are breast and prostate "cancers" that would never be harmful, if we didn't go looking for them, and that treating them leaves people worse off than they were before they even knew they had cancer.

I desperately wanted to grab the cyclist by the shoulders, shake him vigorously, and yell, "Don't you understand that he's just playing with words? Don't you understand 'high-normal' is still normal? You are FINE!" I also desperately wanted him not to get a stress test that could lead him down the garden path to an iatrogenic stroke. How was I going to walk the "you're fine" line with him?

"Look, I can see how distressed you are over this. You look exhausted."

He nodded. "I haven't had a good night's sleep since I moved here; between worrying about what will happen and the side effects of all these damn pills I can barely close my eyes."

"So, you've already felt the downside of 'playing it safe.'"

"No kidding. I'm beginning to think these pills may kill me before that heart attack gets here."

I nodded vigorously. "You may not be far off. Do you know about the idea of a 'number needed to treat' and a 'number needed to harm?'"

The cyclist looked at me blankly.

I continued. "When we give medicines like what you're taking, it's because we know that if we treat enough people with the condition in question, at least one of them will avoid the really bad outcome, like a heart attack, that we're worried about. That number is the number needed to treat. The problem is that it may take a whole lot of people on medication to prevent even one heart attack—and that's the number needed to treat. On the other hand, if we treat enough people, someone is bound to have side effects that are more than just annoying, like a severe allergy. The number of people receiving treatment that virtually guarantees that one person will have a bad side effect is the number needed to harm.

When the number needed to harm is too close to the number needed to treat—or if it is higher—then we're actually harming people, even if the treatment 'works.'" I leaned in further, making sure he looked up to make eye contact. "I know the numbers well enough to know that for people with 'pre-diseases,' the number needed to treat is enormous, but the number needed to harm when you're taking five medications is very small. I just met you, but I really love how dedicated to healthy living you are. The worst thing I could think of doing for you would be something I believe will hurt you for no good reason."

I know this doesn't sound like a real conversation—most people's conversations with the doctor don't go like this. On the other hand, if we're talking about respecting someone's humanity, then respecting both their intelligence and sincere motivation to preserve their health, while also caring enough about them to put the brakes on before we rush them into unnecessary treatments, is part of the deal. As one of the pocket guides I carried when I was a student put it, "Don't just do something—stand there."

At the same time, the cyclist is an unusual situation—a well person who has to be convinced that he is well. Far more often, we run into the opposite—a person with early stage cancer, cholesterol high enough that if you cut the number in half, they'd still be at risk for a stroke, morbid obesity well on its way to destroying both knees by age 35, or blood sugar so elevated that they can't see straight—but who doesn't see the risk, or doesn't believe anything bad will happen to them as a result.

One of the hardest things to do well in medicine is to bring someone into behavior change, without insulting or scaring them. There may be no excuse for degrading someone, or for making them worry unnecessarily—but there is really no excuse for seeing a problem and failing to address it. It violates the most basic understanding of what modern medicine is supposed to be good at, namely finding disease at an earlier stage than was ever possible before and stopping it from progressing, before it gets to the deadly stage. A friend of a friend who's struggled with obesity for years always managed to falsely reassure himself that everything must be fine, because his doctor never mentioned it at their visits.

I know exactly why—his doctor couldn't figure out how to broach the subject, without accidentally saying something that sounded too much like, "You're fat! Lose weight!" As an intern, I was leaving an exam room in my outpatient clinic with my mentor, Russ

Kolarik, when Russ turned to me and said, "You could have said that better." I asked him what he meant, and I'm ashamed still to admit his answer: "She made an offhand remark about how she was concerned about her weight and thought it might be time to do something about it, and you answered, 'Yeah, you could probably stand to lose about 30 pounds.'"

I have spent the last 11 years and counting trying to avoid repeating that mistake. Coming from me, a doctor skinny enough to have once been nicknamed "Scarecrow," it can sound particularly insulting. "How can he possibly know what I'm going through?" I imagine a patient struggling with their weight saying this to themselves, as I prattle on about weight management. Every insulting, shaming comment from a doctor comes along with this same question, really. "How can he possibly know what I'm going through?" asks the woman staying in the homeless shelter, when the doctor who lives in a sprawling suburban house berates her for not keeping up with her medication regimen. "How can she possibly know what I'm going through?"

The problem with imagining these responses is that it's easy to be scared off from asking the hard questions, or naming the obvious problems. If I can already hear the patient saying, "Get back to me when you're perfect," or "When do you suppose I'd have time to do that?" or "What do you know about my life anyway?" what motivation do I have to try? We need language for discussing difficult topics that is both effective and avoids insulting the patient, either by demeaning them or failing to appreciate their circumstances and honor their struggles.

In residency, I was introduced to a technique called "motivational Interviewing," specifically to help discuss smoking behaviors with parents of my pediatric patients. Rather than launching into a diatribe over the evils of overeating or the perils of tobacco, the doctor gathers information ("I see you smoke about 15 cigarettes a day") and then probes the reasons behind the answers ("I'm interested in why you smoke them—what does it do for you?"). Then, the question gets turned around ("Are there any negatives to smoking? Are there things that make you wish you didn't smoke, or that make you hesitate when you pick up your cigarette?"). Only after the patient's own inner dialogue has been explored does the clinician volunteer information ("Your fear about not being able to keep up with your running buddies is spot on—smoking definitely interferes with breathing, and it can really cut into your vital capacity, meaning how much air you can inhale with your deepest breath") that helps to reinforce the patient's own motivation to change behavior.

Motivational interviewing (MI) assumes three things: that the patient wants to be well and healthy, that the patient has the knowledge they need to make changes in their behavior and environment, and that the patient must choose and invest in the plan to change in order to succeed. Patients know already how much they weigh, smoke, drink, and exercise. Whether grudgingly or enthusiastically, most will self-identify the areas that are the greatest threat to their health, essentially inviting me to assist them in making a change. Nearly as many can readily quote me the number for the Quit Line, show me the icon for MyFitnessPal on their phone, or list the hours for the gym they are going to join. MI allows the behavior change conversation to be less like a parent scolding a child and much more like business partners in a brainstorming meeting, or two friends trying to choose the perfect gift for a third.

The problem I run into with MI is that the language often sounds forced; I feel like I'm having an out-of-body experience, and my voice is possessing a stereotyped TV psychologist, someone who never offers opinions of their own and never reveals what they're actually thinking, but on their hidden notepad is writing, "just plain nuts." I mentioned summer camp earlier. The MI sessions often remind me of discussions we would lead at camp that were one giant exercise in dramatic irony, where the counselors knew the point of the discussion ahead of time and tried to guide the conversation of a group of 13-year-olds in exactly the right direction to get them to reach a conclusion that we had already decided upon before the activity even started. MI is meant to level the playing field, to give voice to the patient's preferences, but in doing so, it also reinforces what I think is the dangerous habit of doctors not revealing what they're thinking to the patient.

As a result, even when I'm trying to behave myself and let the patient name the problem, I end up blurting out some very non-MI things. For example, to a mom of a newborn, using formula in the nursery, because her milk isn't in yet, "Oh, you really shouldn't use formula at this age—it causes nipple confusion and can mean your own milk supply is reduced."

It's a constant struggle for me to remember to start the conversation by asking this poor woman who just brought a baby into the world, either with an Olympian effort or by having abdominal surgery, whether she wants to breastfeed, and how earnestly and for how long. I repeatedly forget to sound out how much knowledge the woman has about breastmilk and how to get it from her own body to the baby's, even though she may have breastfed three previous children for a year and a half each.

With older children, I may want to honor parents' own ideas of how to solve their child's sleep problems, or explain the behavior issues in school, or discuss their readiness to potty train, but the urge to just hand them a copy of the Ferber book, refer them to the school psychologist, or tell them not to use M&Ms as a reward is just too strong. For a doctor who doesn't really believe in paternalistic medicine (telling patients what to do), I tell people what to do an awful lot. "Don't smoke in your house." "Make sure your child knows your address and phone number before school." "You really shouldn't give him juice to drink in a bottle—he's too old and it's terrible for his teeth."

The same urge strikes me with adults as well. Needing to find a way out of my knee-jerk response of giving people advice they may not want, and answering questions that haven't been asked of me yet, I've spent the last several years looking for language that works for me to make the interaction more of a dialogue and less of a speech.

Healing People, Not Patients

One of my teachers challenges patients on behaviors that she thinks need changing by saying, "I'm confused." It is a way to start a conversation, when a patient's behavior and a patient's concerns seem to be running counter to each other. "I'm confused" is the response when a diabetic patient tells her he is eating better, and then lists a daily menu that includes mashed potatoes, Pepsi, two sandwiches, and a plate of spaghetti. "I'm confused" is a subtle way of letting the patient critique themself—contrasting the way they want to perceive the situation with what is actually going on and waiting for the patient to realize the contradiction. "You're right, doctor, I need to do a better job of controlling my carbs—and here I thought just 'cause I wasn't eating fried foods, I was doing a good job." There is a bit of embarrassment, sheepishness really, but because the patient has called themself out, it is less than if the doctor had berated or belittled him.

I've also experimented with starting from a stance of concern: "I'm worried about what will happen to your health if you keep smoking." With a long-time patient with whom a good relationship exists, I can even go a step further: "Harold, you know how devastated I'd be if you had a heart attack. I don't know what I'd do without you coming in to my office every three months and making the same awful jokes with the receptionists."

With time, I earn the right to open up and parlay the trust and intimacy I've developed with a patient into the ability to be frank. Even when I don't have the luxury of the comfortable old relationship, I can still adopt this stance. That caring begins the minute I meet someone. "I know we've just met, but you came to me because you were looking to get control of your health and live a better life, as you're entering your 60s. I'm so glad you did, but I have to tell you that I'm worried about whether you'll be able to meet that goal, if you don't start getting some regular exercise."

Once I've gotten my concerns laid on the table, then it's easier for me to conduct a motivational interview. I can compare my concerns with the patient's, and sound out readiness to change, without feeling like I'm playing mind games. Often, by doing this, I end up uncovering the real obstacle to behavior change: a 20-year-old is trying to lose weight but lives with grandma, who feeds her to show love. A child is spending too much time in front of the TV because the family has no car, and the nearest playground is too far away for them to walk. An IV drug user is trying to quit, but has housing that directly overlooks the bar where they have always bought their drugs. The real goals become clear—in all of these cases, housing is the real problem and has to be addressed, before any behavior change can take place.

Other times, I can lay out my concerns all I want. One patient, a Korea era Navy vet, always makes the same joke when I mention his smoking. "Doctor, I don't drink anymore, and I don't chase women, because I forget what to do with 'em when I catch up to 'em." Another regularly asks me why he's so short of breath, even though he has a normal stress test and doesn't have asthma. He doesn't argue when I tell him that it's related to his substantial obesity—he only argues when I tell him he has to give up his donuts. "Ain't gonna happen!" he laughs and smiles.

I've known both of these men for years, and it helps me going in to know that I'm going to make one plea, get the same answer I've come to expect, and not get frustrated at the status quo. The illness is hypothetical, and I'm trying to get these two to take actions whose success will be that nothing happens. Giving up the donuts and cigarettes, though? That's not hypothetical—that's real, and it's a non-starter.

The conversations are even harder, both on an emotional and a skill level, when the illness is already ongoing and possibly terminal. For the last 10 years, when I'm not seeing patients in the office, I've been involved in a project called Closure: Changing Expectations for End of Life. Closure started when the folks I work for at the Jewish Healthcare Foundation in Pittsburgh realized that they were constantly hearing stories about people's experiences with friends and relatives who were dying of illness—and that the stories were even more awful than one might imagine, being that all of them ended in death.

Underlying all of this heartache is the perception that death is optional, something that happens to other, unfortunate people, but not to us. Long conversations and policy meetings could take place on the topic of aging and caring for the very elderly, and yet the word "death" wouldn't even merit a mention.

It's a common shared delusion in American medicine—the idea that the patient is invincible, and the medical system is omnipotent, and infallible. The old joke runs that Mr. Jones is dying of leukemia and lapses into kidney failure, necessitating a nephrology consult. The consultants come by and pronounce Mr. Jones an excellent candidate for dialysis, and if they can just get his kidneys a little rest, they'll be good as new. The oncologists are thrilled, since they have been certain all along that one more round of treatment will have him in remission for sure.

The next morning the oncology team arrives at Mr. Jones' bedside to find him missing. They frantically hunt down the nurse, who calmly informs them that Mr. Jones died peacefully during the night.

"Died? That's impossible! He was just about to turn the corner!" they all shout. They demand to know where he is, and the nurse shrugs and directs them to the morgue. Forgoing the elevator, they race down the stairs to the basement and shout at the clerk that they need to know which drawer Mr. Jones is in, and fast. The clerk, barely raising his eyes from his computer screen, indicates drawer #34. The oncology fellow seizes the metal handle, yanks on it with all her might, and slides out the gurney, only to find it empty, except for a small scrap of paper on which is scrawled:

"Back in four hours—gone to dialysis."

It would be funnier, if we didn't behave exactly like this much of the time, whether we are treating cancer, end-stage organ failure, massive brain trauma, or the last throes of dementia. In residency, I gradually came to view certain treatments I saw being ordered on patients I was helping to care for as the medical equivalent of red jerseys in a Star Trek episode: marks of impending death, a sort of foreshadowing funded by Medicare. Granulocyte transfusions, drips of the cardiac drug nesiritide, continuous dialysis, antibiotic regimens greater than three drugs, which included both an antifungal and an antiviral—all of these were harbingers of doom, a virtual promise I would be back in that room pronouncing death before too long.

These treatments were signs of one of our greatest failures in medicine, the failure to be honest with ourselves and our patients that some sicknesses do actually end in death. By treating death as a complication, rather than the ultimate outcome of all life, we delude ourselves into thinking that everyone can be saved at any time. Even when we acknowledge the eventuality of death, we think it's a lot further off than it really is. One famous study reviewed charts from the day before patients' deaths and found that the average predicted life expectancy in those notes was six months. We can't even recognize impending death when the patient is already on their deathbed.

When we do recognize death, we do a terrible job conveying it to the patient and family. We use language that hedges our bets, that backs away from using the word death, which obscures the fact that the patient is becoming inexorably sicker. For this reason I had one attending in residency who took the unusual step of teaching the residents how to make a phone call to a family member. "If the patient is very sick," he said, "don't begin the phone call by saying, 'He's not doing well.' They will hear the 'well' instead of the 'not.' Say, 'He's doing poorly.' There can't be a mistake made there."

There were months in residency where this was all I did: pediatric ICU, cardiac ICU, medical ICU. I shuttled back and forth from conference rooms filled with haggard family members to bedside; elbow-deep in blood and wires. One week in the pediatric unit five children died, all but one of foreseeable causes. It was during that very week, in fact, that a family sat quietly by the side of their critically ill daughter, almost unrecognizable, when I thought of how she had looked on her first admission the previous summer, and resolutely told me they were expecting a miracle. Outside the room an exasperated pastor turned to me and said words that I have never forgotten: "Sometimes, the miracle is heaven."

In the midst of learning to grapple with this level of medical futility, my grandfather fell ill. Really, he had been falling ill for five years, since suffering a heart attack a mere eight days after my aunt Janet, his younger daughter, died of multiple myeloma when she was not yet 50. Gramp was a medical miracle since birth, having been born with an imperforate anus and needing multiple corrective bowel and urinary surgeries by the time he was six weeks old. I'm told that a distant cousin who trained at Johns Hopkins medical school once heard Gramp's case presented in his surgical residency, so unusual had it been. Years later, when I was entering medical school, he survived early stage colon cancer. The blow of losing a child, however, proved too much for his heart, and it broke. He recovered from the heart attack, but was never the same. A little slower, a little less sure of himself behind the wheel, despite a lifetime traversing the highways of the tri-state area as an insurance salesman. A little less able to hold his own when bickering with my grandmother, something they had perfected in 50-plus years of marriage.

The month that I was on the cardiac ICU, however, was different. I got a page during rounds one morning, only to discover that it wasn't even from within the same hospital where I was working and had nothing to do with any of the patients on my service. It was my own PCP, covering hospital rounds for the group where both Gramp and I got our medical care, calling to tell me that Gramp had been admitted, and there were some things we needed to discuss.

The problems had piled up too high. The miraculous surgery done in the 1920s had exceeded its warranty, and the crazy, re-routed plumbing had begun prolapsing through places it shouldn't, failing to drain urine properly, and getting infected. Overwhelmed by the pressure, his kidneys failed, and he started dialysis, never his idea of the way he wanted to live, but something about which he felt he had no choice. With that underway, he began to have the usual complications: one week the fistula was infected, another it clotted, another they removed too much fluid or not enough potassium, and he felt sick for days after treatment. Now, he was hospitalized with another fistula issue, but there was something else wrong, a pain in his upper right abdomen that wouldn't relent.

"There are three spots on the liver on the ultrasound," Anthony explained, "and let's be honest, I'd be shocked if they were anything other than cancer. Are we sure his colon cancer was in remission?"

I assured him that it was; my grandmother had been perseverating on the normal results of the last colonoscopy for months. But, that meant that some other malign process was spreading into his liver.

"He's not going to want to do anything about this," I told Anthony over the phone. "When the colon cancer was diagnosed, he swore to me he'd never do chemotherapy, and he was true to his word then. He's a lot sicker now, so I can't imagine he'd change his mind."

I was right. Rather than rush into a decision in the hospital, Gramp went home, his dialysis fistula repaired for now, and on a chilly, rainy January Saturday afternoon, I went from the cardiac ICU directly to his tiny living room in the senior high-rise, where he now lived. Medical supplies and clutter overwhelmed the space, tangible evidence of his declining health and independence.

I was brutally honest that afternoon, but only because he asked me to be, and because no one could BS my grandfather and get away with it.

"How likely is it that these spots were cancer?" he asked. Almost certain, I told him.

Did he want to know for sure? "What would that take, finding out?" When I told him a liver biopsy, we were done. Nothing was worth that. Especially when it became clear that the best case scenario, metastatic colon cancer that had somehow escaped detection on the colonoscopy, would only allow him to live a few months longer, and then only with the not-going-to-do-it chemotherapy, than the worst case, namely an "unknown primary."

"It's hell getting old," he sighed, for the first of what would be many times over the next few weeks.

"What about dialysis?" I asked.

"What happens if I stop?" he wanted to know.

Stopping dialysis is actually one of the most painless ways to die, if you are nearing the end of life. Toxins, which the kidneys, or the artificial kidneys that we call dialysis machines, normally clear from the blood stream, build up over a period of a week or two. Eventually, they reach levels where they begin to drug the patient into a quiet, confused (though itchy) stupor, generally sapping consciousness a couple days before the electrolyte imbalance stops the heart. He took this in slowly, pondered it, and decided he'd keep going, for now.

A little over a week later he got lost driving the half-mile across the bridge to the dialysis center. My mother found him confused and frightened in a parking lot about a block from his destination. He never went back. Hospice arrived with a hospital bed the very next day, and he followed an almost textbook course from that point until he died, 10 days later. The last thing he said to me, besides reminding me again that it was hell getting old, was, "I'll be 85 and a half years old on Thursday." He died Friday at 3 a.m.

Maybe two years later, I was eating dinner with friends and extended family, when the topic turned to end of life, and I mentioned Gramp's decision. My friend's mother turned to me and said simply, "I remember. He was my hero."

It's paradoxical for us to think of someone being a hero because they stop fighting, but that's not what she meant. He was a hero, because he stared into the face of the thing we all fear the most, and walked right toward it, without hesitation. But, when I consider how he got to that point, I think of how lucky he had to be in order to be able to make the decision he wanted to make, to exit this world on his terms. He had to have a grandson who was graduating a medical residency, who was emotionally able to sit down and have a gut-wrenching conversation with a man he adored, and who was willing to be frank enough to say, "Gramp, you're dying, and there is nothing much we can do to stop it from happening very soon. How do you want to deal with that?"

Closure is supposed to prepare people like me and people like Gramp to have the hardest conversation of their lives. It's meant to remove the mystery surrounding death and dying, and the mystique surrounding "heroic medical treatment" that often serves only to prolong suffering. It's meant to allow people as much agency to write the last chapter of their life stories as they have to write the chapters about marriage, career, or personal passions. Most of all, it is meant to turn death back into a natural event in the course of life.

Teaching the Closure curriculum has been a passion of mine ever since, having brought these discussions to houses of worship, libraries, elder-college courses, fellow professionals, and even an undergraduate religious studies course. By and by, I've realized what makes these discussions so incredibly difficult.

In the end of life community, we will often refer to people as either "getting it" or "not getting it," meaning people that do or don't understand the basic premise that dying is natural, inevitable, and cannot always be postponed, without an unbearable cost to the patient and family. But, what happens when someone "gets it" and decides they don't care?

We sat on a cigarette-burned sofa in a dimly-lit living room, and Harriet said, "Doctor, I am angry with you. I haven't felt comfortable talking with you for the last few months. The last time you saw me, you told me we weren't going to bother with my mammogram this year. I felt like you were giving up on me."

I felt, once again, like I was an unsure, second-guessing resident, just as I had been when we met four years earlier. I remembered the conversation well. It happened after two near-death hospitalizations for respiratory failure. Afterward, she canceled (at my urging) a long-awaited trip to visit an old friend out-of-state (this is apparently a bad habit of mine); it was clear to both of us that traveling that far could be the last trip she took.

The next time she saw me she told me, not for the first time, that she wouldn't be surprised if she didn't live out a year; I'm not sure if she meant until New Year's or her next birthday. It was just after she said this that the subject of mammograms came up. Knowing how she felt, and knowing how delicately balanced all of her multiple, serious medical problems were, I had to agree. To me, that meant that she was not likely to survive long enough for anything she saw on a mammogram to do her additional harm. Harriet made no secret of her hatred for hospitals and doctors' offices (mine included), and I did not intend to put her through a test she didn't need.

Then, three months passed, and it appeared I had been wrong. She had felt a lump before that previous visit, and she wanted—still wanted, even now, feeling even worse than she had then—that mammogram.

I wrote the prescription; I don't think she ever used it. She died three months later, after a week and a half in hospice that her husband later called "the most pleasant hospital stay she had during this whole mess."

Sometime later, I was teaching a Closure seminar about having an open, honest conversation about death, trying to break out of the Brighton Beach Memoirs superstition that if you say it, it might happen to you. The discussion ended with a personal story from one of the participants who was dying—her words, and her doctors'—of a liver abscess two years prior, only to come back "escaped to tell thee" like one of the messengers coming to Job. What had saved her was a surgery that had one chance in a hundred of succeeding, and a much higher chance of leaving her dead on the operating table. Why was she undergoing the surgery? Her daughter insisted that, "If she's going to die anyway, why don't you operate? What have you got to lose?"

It's hard to argue with the outcome of this previously dying woman, who walked into the room under her own power, sat attentively in a lecture and discussion for an hour, and chose this moment to articulately tell the story of how reports of her death had been greatly exaggerated. Her daughter said: "If she's dying anyway ..." Eyes wide open, knowing the likely outcome, she took a chance, the only one she had, to bring a previously well woman back from death's door.

To people like Harriet or the woman in my lecture, our frank, nuanced conversations about death send the message, "We are not going to try to save you anymore." That's not what we mean, but it's what they hear. Never mind that we are trying to save them—save them from tremendous suffering that may actually shorten their lifespan, without doing anything to improve the life in that span, as we know often happens with lung cancer patients. It sounds too much like the "hanging crepe" approach: "You're dying—get your affairs in order, there's nothing more we can do for you."

To make matters worse, we often can't make up our minds about whether someone is actually dying or not. Once upon a time, perhaps, doctors were better at prognosticating, more certain—except that the certainty was death. Old editions of medical textbooks contained long sections on the "natural history" of each disease, including how long people were likely to survive and what the stages of progression toward death might be—often the stages which gave diseases their very colorful nicknames, like "consumption" or "lockjaw." As we grew better at curing, we grew worse at predicting—almost as if our newfound knowledge had clouded the crystal ball. Once everyone knew how the story would end. Now—who knows?

We hate saying it—it makes us look foolish, almost incompetent. Our patients are desperate for answers, and to their most fundamental questions we have none. The answers that we do give are often non-answers, like "I don't practice prophecy, I practice medicine." Other times, they are deliberately vague, like, "somewhere between 6 and 24 months," or even obfuscate the truth, like "the median three-year disease free survival rate with acceptable neurological outcome and minimal residual functional deficits is ..."

Worse, on occasion, we give confident answers—knowing full well that we have no way of knowing what the answer is. Every doctor I know has a story in which that misplaced confidence convinces an exhausted terminal cancer patient to endure another round of "salvage" chemotherapy, thinking that a cure may have been found, when even the prescribing doctor harbors no hope of success. Yet, just as many doctors have a story of the patient who is given six months to live, and tells this to a large audience—of mourners at the doctor's funeral 20 years later.

Even with patients who are not at the end of life, there is still much that we don't know. Who knows if you and your wife will get pregnant this time around, but I have seen it work with many couples, and I know how desperately you want it, and if it fails, I will not give up trying with you. Who knows if this cold will go away by the weekend, but it usually does, and if not, here's my number, please call. Who knows if the back surgery will finally heal your pain—here are some reasons why it might and here are some reasons why not. What do you think you want to do?

The problem is when we react to the uncertainty by failing to be honest with our patients about how unclear the picture is, or by defaulting to exhaustive workups and full-bore treatment, which they gladly accept, because they think we know what we're doing. When we do become certain that death, or permanent disability, or continued infertility will be the outcome, we stop so abruptly that the patient cannot help but feel abandoned.

Words have tremendous power in medicine, as much as many of our medicines and surgeries. When those interventions go wrong, we rake the offending physician over the coals in a conference known as morbidity and mortality—M&M for short.

I think it's time we start a new conference—the F-in-M conference, for foot in mouth. I would be willing to bet it saves as many lives—and relationships—as the other one.

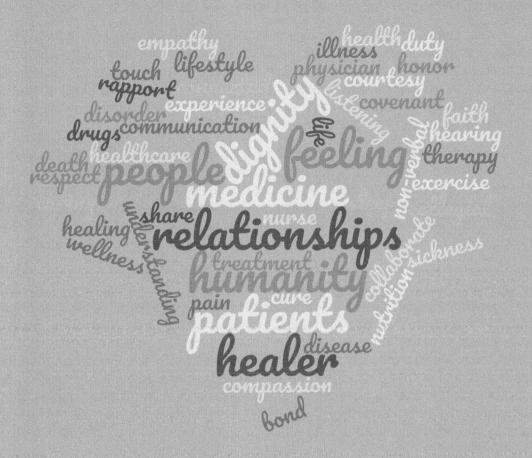

CHAPTER 5

Words Unspoken

It was 3 a.m. on my last night on call in an intensive care unit, the same month I had learned that my grandfather was dying. As a fourth year resident, I'd spent a year of my life caring for critically-ill people of all ages in brightly-lit rooms where time is of the essence, and yet time never seems to pass. It had left many marks on me, few of them visible.

At that particular moment, however, I was engaged in removing one of the visible marks—a large blood stain on the left side of my white lab coat, just at waist level. I had just discovered the magical powers of hydrogen peroxide, and was in the process of restoring my coat to presentability before rounds the next morning. I couldn't undo the damage done by witnessing so many agonizing deaths, or by realizing I was losing my grandfather, but I *could* get out that damn spot.

The coat is one of the core symbols of my profession in many people's minds. It is an outward symbol of the link between modern medicine and modern science: the same lab coat worn behind the lab bench serves to identify the scientist at the bedside. In much the same way, I imagine the long robes worn by medieval physicians in paintings I have seen from that period probably evoked images of the contemporary clergy, in an era where healing was felt to be more in the hands of God than genomics.

Doctors and their coats have a complicated relationship, and that relationship impacts the relationship between them and the patients for whom they care. Years ago, people inherently trusted their doctors more than any other profession, with the possible exception of clergy. I don't think there is the same level of innocent trust in any profession today, and medicine is no different. Hardly a popular magazine hits the stand today without an article claiming to have information that "your doctor won't tell you about." We have tarnished our own profession through our relationships with industry, our failure to regulate ourselves in a way that removes the bad apples from the barrel, and our continued hesitation to solve the crisis that leaves millions in our country and billions around the world without access to the level of care we are capable of providing.

Yet, there is still some special aura about the medical profession, and the white coat may enhance that aura. There is purity about the white coat, perhaps because of its message of scientific objectivity and lack of prejudice that restores some of medicine's mystique. At the same time, as a white garment, it fits the cultural message of other white garments. Brides wear white dresses at their weddings to symbolize their purity, though the truth of that symbol is tarnished in an era of second marriages and commonplace premarital sex. Perhaps, as the reputation of medicine has fallen, the white lab coat has taken the same sort of devaluation as the white wedding gown.

Even with this, the coat is still held up as a symbol. My medical school, and many others in the country, inducts the incoming students into the profession by holding a White Coat Ceremony on the Sunday immediately before the start of orientation. Other schools, like the physician assistant program where I teach, do a similar ceremony at graduation. For many people, the first time they meet their classmates is in this context, as the faculty of the school of medicine address the students, and one-by-one place the physical and symbolic burden of the coat upon the students' shoulders. Students who are to be second- or third-generation physicians often have their mothers or grandfathers "coat" them, much as a graduating student will choose to have their mentor present their hood or diploma.

Four years later, entering residency, students again receive their white coats; in all but a few places, the new coats are now full-length coats, instead of the jacket-length student coats. The residents will often point out that the new coats finally cover their backsides, perhaps giving them confidence in their knowledge, so that they no longer have to worry about covering their behinds when they speak. White garments, of any length, also symbolize transition, wiping the slate clean and starting over—with a freshly minted degree, a new level of confidence and authority, and often in a completely new location, thanks to the vagaries of the Match program.

Unfortunately, the white coat carries the baggage of negative connotation as well. I recently read a brilliant ode to a white coat written by a young female resident. For her, the coat was a symbol for everything from the cluttered armamentarium of scarce supplies she carried in it, to her deteriorating married life, to her gnawing sense of inadequacy, to the many stains of failure, real and imagined, that the coat carried. I did my own residency under the guidance of a program director who shared with us that he hadn't worn a coat since the day he left residency, because it carried with it all the frustration he had felt as a resident.

White coats are frightening. Studies have shown that children are more likely to be frightened at the doctor if their pediatrician or family doctor wears a white coat over her cartoon necktie. My adult patients don't have it any easier: they suffer from "white-coat hypertension," a malady wherein the mere sight of me decked out in Ivory Snow pure polyester sends their blood pressure through the roof. "I swear, Doctor Weinkle, when I took my blood pressure in the pharmacy this weekend, it was perfect!" Of course, it continues to be a problem when I'm not wearing my coat; maybe I just make people nervous.

Are patients worried about the men, from the old novelty song, "in the little white coats who are coming to take me away?" The Cuckoo's Nest sinister connotation that the coat carries is so powerful that as med students on the inpatient psychiatric rotation, we were forbidden to put our coats on (or wear our ID badges, or ties, or anything that gave the patients a reason to be angry with us, or a place to grab us). The coat puts up a wall between the patient and doctor, creating a relationship that is unequal, even threatening.

It's not just paranoid schizophrenics who get antsy around the doctor wearing the coat:

Me: "Mr. Brown! Great to see you. It's been a really long time, hasn't It?"

Brown: "Well, I hadn't been taking care of my diabetes real well. Missed my medications a lot. I guess I was embarrassed to come see you; I knew you'd be mad at me."

What is it about the doctor-patient relationship that makes patients behave like children about to be scolded by their parents, when they haven't heard the doctor's advice? At least some of it is the power differential—represented, if not actually created, by the white coat.

I'm not a fashion aficionado; it is words, not threads, that get my attention. So, it's humbling to think that all the care I put into choosing my words, in saying, "You're fine" or "You're dying," with just the right balance of honesty and compassion, can be overshadowed by what I'm wearing. But, it's true.

Just as easily as people can be intimidated or ashamed by the white coat, they can be impressed as well. There's a whole body of white-coat research, and it turns out that patients actually perceive doctors wearing white coats, as well as semi-formal dress, like men's ties, as being more compassionate *and more competent*, even before they open their mouths. Too much starch may make a doctor appear distant, cold, or intimidating. On the other hand, too much slouch makes them appear incapable of treating so much as a hangnail.

One of my long-time Nepali translators always complements how "smart" I look, when I wear a tie. One day in the middle of winter, he and I were scheduled to work together on our mobile unit, which is well-intentioned but poorly insulated. It was cold and snowing outside, so I dressed for the weather, in a collarless shirt and a sweater. When Pancham saw me, he hung his head in disappointment. "The people," he sighed, meaning the folks he translates for, "like how nice you dress," meaning in a shirt and tie. Turn up the heat …

Suddenly, my office manager's good faith effort to boost employee morale with a dress-down day turns into a moral dilemma. What impression does dressing down leave on the patients? I work in primary care, so the classic nightmare scenario of an emergency nurse wearing a clown costume while informing parents that their child has died is very unlikely. But, how seriously will my patients who have never seen ice before they came to the US be able to take my words, if I'm wearing my Mark Andre-Fleury hockey jersey? Will my smiling, yoga-devoted friend Prasad think I am disrespecting him, if I ditch my tie and wool trousers, and wear jeans and a polo shirt because it's too hot outside for my usual wardrobe? Do casual Fridays really tell the Friday patients that they don't count as much as the ones the rest of the week, because we're all in too much of a hurry to get out of there for the weekend?

The answer is that by standardizing the dress code, even for dress-down days, we create almost an alternate uniform, like throwback jerseys in professional sports, or Osler ties and scarves on Fridays for the physicians at Johns Hopkins. On the other hand, how we solved the problem is less important than the fact that it exists, that the words we exchange are spoken in a context that includes what we are wearing.

It includes what the patient is wearing—or isn't wearing—too. We're accustomed to thinking about patient gowns as a necessary evil, one that enables us to hook up monitors in the hospital or conduct an effective skin exam or Pap smear in the office. But, as someone who has more than my fair share of strange-looking moles, I have undergone a lot of whole-body skin exams. My old dermatologist used paper gowns. By the time the exam ended I would be down to nothing but boxer shorts and a scarf of shredded paper. Considering I was talking with someone who was supposed to be a colleague (and whom I knew socially), it was hard to muster up my dignity again until I got dressed.

Street clothes definitely get in the way of physical exams—it is really hard to do an abdominal exam on a woman in a long dress, or a knee exam on a person wearing jeans, or a testicular exam on a man in tight trousers and briefs, who is too embarrassed to unzip all the way. The dilemma with patient gowns is this—how much of someone's nakedness do I need to uncover, and for how long, to really do a good job? Is the exam even necessary? And if I leave them sitting in an embarrassing, degrading, humiliating state for longer than needed, how much does it matter that I am speaking with caring, compassionate words?

The sobering realization that "semi-private" rooms, too-short hospital gowns, and "standard" physical exam practices could be undermining all of the carefully chosen words I use has had a strange effect on me. Each time I reach for a gown for a patient to put on, I debate whether it's really needed—and exactly what I am asking them to remove when they put it on. I now consider dignity shorts (a specialty garment made to be worn during colonoscopies, which, if you ask most people, are the ultimate *indignity*) to be a fair topic for ethical discussion. If I'm going to value a patient's human dignity equally with my own, then I don't want them to feel like I do after my mole checks …

Even if both of us are fully dressed, however, there is plenty I can do that can devalue well-chosen words—beginning with the *way* I say them.

About six months ago, I made a technological breakthrough—I finally got the clock to appear on my computer screen at the bottom of the electronic medical record window. This was crucial, because it turns out that no matter what I was saying to a patient, if I looked up at the clock while I was doing it, they heard only one thing: "I have more important things to do than talking to you." It's no secret that doctors are under enormous time pressure, and that *not* looking at the clock will lead to me running late and disrespecting the *next* patient. But, there was something about that obvious glance at the wall, away from both the patient and the screen where I was taking notes, that conveyed to them that nothing else mattered but time.

Body language like this can make or break a conversation. I'm an efficient note-taker and fast typist and find myself able to do so much more for my patients when I write my notes while I am seeing them. They talk, I type, then I talk and type at the same time as I'm explaining myself. The problem, of course, is that this keeps my eyes glued to the computer screen. I use a laptop, so at least I'm facing the patient, but my gaze is on the device, not their face. Before I got the laptop, it was worse—the desktop monitors are against the wall, and I would have to literally look over my shoulder if I wanted to see the patient while also sitting in front of the computer.

I'm a huge fan of electronic records, ever since my days as a med student, when I would waste hours waiting for the file clerk in the radiology department at the VA to locate an x-ray, and the time my wife changed medical practices because she had an appointment in one office, but her paper chart was in the other office. I would never go back. But, at the same time, I know my patients feel like they need my eye contact to tell me that I'm hearing them, instead of just charting obsessively so I can get paid for my time. I know this, because I hear their complaints about other doctors they see: "He never looked at me." "She cared more about that damn computer screen than about me." Asking all the right questions in the first half of the visit does not make up for the awkward silence in the second half because I can't find the right ICD-10 code in the system.

Fortunately, we've made some conscious adjustments in my office to make this problem better. Most of the providers have now gone over to laptops, including the medical assistants, and the new office doesn't even have desktop computers, so that the provider can always face the patient. The new laptops flip inside-out to tablets with styluses. If I can ever figure out how to get the thing to work efficiently, it will be like going back to my med school days, when I could sit on the edge of the patient's bed and take notes by hand, while maintaining eye contact. And ultimately, I have learned to free myself a little from the tyranny of the computer and just stop typing for a while, whenever I need to listen more intensely, or whenever I need to explain something—because who can talk with their hands and type at the same time?

For that matter, the act of talking with my hands itself, and all of the other things I do to lend feeling to my words, turns out to be a critical component of the medical conversation as well. It's not a secret that there are "right things" to say in certain situations: "I'm sorry for your loss," when we hear about the death of a loved one, for example. Sure, there are many doctors who forget to say even that; they gloss over it as if they didn't even hear the person mention their mother's passing. But, it's just as easy, sometimes, to acknowledge a passing in passing, so mechanically that it almost wasn't worth saying.

I've done it myself far too often. The patient will be explaining a trying set of circumstances and say something like, "and then of course my mother died of cancer last month." Almost before I can stop myself I have said, "I'm sorry for your loss," in the same tone I just used to say, "Your x-ray result isn't back yet."

Healing People, Not Patients

The patient's life changed irrevocably last month. Sure, I need to offer condolences—but not in a rote, by-the-book fashion. The patient can hear the script. They can recognize the rehearsed lines. What they need is evidence that the doctor is not phoning it in. They need presence, and we need a way to provide it for them that requires more than just words.

About a year ago, I heard the eulogy of a much more senior colleague, in which he was described as "the kind of person who listened with both ears." I immediately thought of my pulmonology instructors at Children's Hospital, who all carry stethoscopes with one bell for each side of the chest, but I knew that wasn't what the speaker meant. This late giant of medicine had been empathetic, caring, and devoted his full attention to hearing the patient's story. But, as the tales of his career spun on, I realized a different meaning to the phrase, "listen with both ears."

As important as listening to the patient may be, we can only afford to devote one ear to listening to her. The other ear, the one this gentleman used so well, needs to be turned inward, so we can hear ourselves. Not only the content of our words but their tone, their prosody, their connotations. We need to detect sarcasm, anger, and especially boredom and disinterest.

When I utter a phrase like, "Sorry for your loss," in a completely offhand manner, that second ear needs to stop me cold, and make me present in the moment again. I need to lock eyes with the patient, offer visible support, and delve deeper. What happened? Was she ill long? How is this affecting you? Even if it is not medically relevant to the patient's diagnosis, it is essential to the relationship for her to know that I care enough to share in her grief in more than just a cursory way.

Since realizing this, having a conversation has become a totally different experience for me, especially in the clinic. As I speak, I am simultaneously editing my words, either to correct them or try for better the next time. Did I just take a good open-ended question and turn it into a closed-ended, "either-or" question? I have noticed this tendency over and again—try though I might, I cannot just leave a question open to interpretation, I guess for fear that the patient will misunderstand it. The second ear has helped me hear that—now if I only had a second tongue to keep the first one from speaking so much.

Did I just steamroll over someone sharing really important emotional data? Once, about five years ago, I couldn't get my own head together before entering the room. Even though the patient had written on the intake sheet that he was feeling depressed, I decided to table the conversation about emotions and told the patient as much, even saying that it was because I couldn't handle it that day. I spent close to a year repairing that relationship. Again, the second ear hears when I am reacting from my gut instead of my heart or my head, as well as when I am not choosing my words carefully or thinking about their impact.

Did I just add to someone's confusion with my "explanation" of their problems? I've said already how the language we speak in medicine is only loosely connected to English or any other language spoken by real people. Yet, we are so steeped in it that it is perfectly natural for us to say words like "idiopathic," "iatrogenic," or "myocardial infarction," and not realize that our patients have no idea what these mean. We don't realize that when we give one label to a condition that another physician has called by another name, we don't reassure—we make people feel sicker.

I actually have patients who begin to doubt that their doctors are telling them the truth, because they don't hear different words for the same diagnosis—they hear a completely different story. The confusion we sow doesn't just make they less clear on what's going on, it makes them less able to trust us. The second ear hears what a layman hears and alerts us to speak with more clarity and consistency, and to explain how our explanation fits with our colleagues' explanations.

Ultimately, however, our best chosen words are not tested by what we're wearing when we say them, or what tone of voice we use to deliver them. They are tested by what we do, or don't do to follow them up. Medicine these days talks a good game. Every ad, every brochure, every practice trumpets their compassion, their "patient-centered" approach, their comprehensiveness. For all the talk, however, it is our deeds that are the proof of the pudding.

Most medical conversations end with a "what now?" stage. As the encounter ends, it can feel to a patient as if they are stepping back out into the jungle, venturing out into the unknown, only marginally more sure of what to do than they were when they came in. What is going to happen, wonders the young mother, when my child wakes up coughing and won't go back to sleep again tonight? What will I do tomorrow when I once again wake up with a headache, and this new medicine doesn't work, but I need to go to work? Where do I go when I cannot bear the discomfort any longer? Do I have diabetes, or don't I?

When these questions arise at the end of a visit, my tendency is to be incredibly reassuring. Don't worry, I'm here for you. If this doesn't work, we can try something else. You can always call. But, is that really true, or is there going to be three months of radio silence, until this patient shows up again, even closer to the end of her rope than she was before, about to be fired or perhaps out of work, believing that her child has some life-threatening disease, or convinced he himself is about to die of a heart attack day after tomorrow?

I've thought about the opposite approach, the "say little and do much" attitude, but the reassurance of words does help to calm the fear. The easy out of setting, and then exceeding, low expectations doesn't work when someone has already put their life in your hands. On the other hand, the higher the expectation, the harder it is to make good on it.

Healing People, Not Patients

I'm a terrible correspondent. As a friend, I've regrettably lost touch with some of the people I've been closest with—and been blessed to choose such wonderful friends that they allow me to rekindle those friendships many years later. My patients don't have that luxury of allowing me to disappear on them for years at a time (the ones that *do* have that luxury usually disappear on *me*). They have pressing needs that require my attention and counsel today and tomorrow. Of all the complaints that people have about today's medical system, perhaps the most damning criticism is the feeling of being abandoned—and the highest praise I hear is heaped on my colleagues who never abandon someone in their hour of need.

The problem is that it's easy to let these well-intentioned promises slip away from me. Even very concrete tasks, like a driver's permit form, certification of medical leave from work, or a signature on a school physical, can always fall to the bottom of the queue when we're busy. But, some of our promises are more intricate and difficult to complete than that. A pledge to check in on someone in their hour of need. A commitment to advocate with a specialist, or an insurer, or an employer, with whom the patient cannot reason. A research project to find out what cutting edge treatments are on the horizon so this patient does not need to give up hope. Have I held myself out as a superhero, only to disappoint?

In residency, I would obsessively make check boxes on 5"x8" index cards to keep track of everything I had to do for my patients—check lab results, call consultants, write discharge orders. These days, I am using my Microsoft Outlook task list to do the same thing with maintaining relationships. "Mary, hold on one second. I agree we should really keep a close record of whether you feel any better on this new medication. I'm setting myself a reminder to call you two weeks from Thursday to check in. *pause* There. Now, it's on my 'to-do' list. You'll hear from me, I promise." Sometimes, I get busy. Sometimes, I forget—and the disappointment is not lost on me.

It seems obvious that promises should be kept, that words should be backed up with deeds. But, I have sent patients who speak minimal English for diagnostic testing at hospitals that adorn their entrances with signs that say "welcome" in multiple languages—only to have them sent away by technicians who did not bother to call a translator when they could not convey the instructions in English. I have spoken with newly delivered mothers who were promised natural childbirth and a trial of labor after a C-section—only to have the on-call obstetrician tell them, "I don't do *those*," and bundle them off to the operating suite. I have also cared for patients pumped full of hope by consultants, who tell them that they are perfect candidates for a new imaging technique or a specialized surgery—only to be dismissed as patients, without warning, a week later, when insurance, ego, personality, or some other circumstance made it inconvenient to continue.

Healing People, Not Patients

So, every time someone thanks me for going the extra mile for them, for making one more phone call or reading one more research article on their behalf, I wonder who else I have let down, what other commitments I have forgotten about in the process. I have a sneaking feeling that those broken promises are stains on my coat that the peroxide cannot remove.

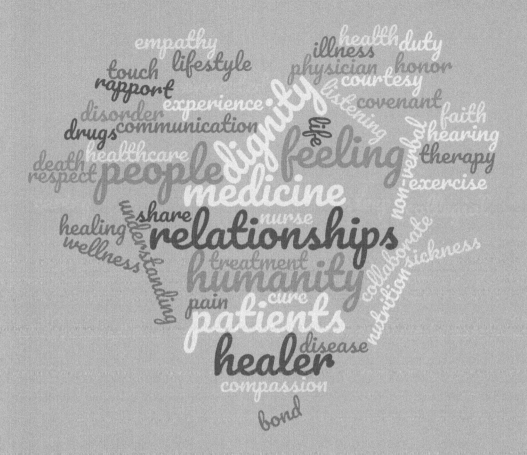

CHAPTER 6

In This Together

I work with a medical assistant, whom I've nicknamed Radar. I grew up watching reruns of the TV show *M*A*S*H*, and one of the greatest recurring bits in the show was the way Corporal Walter "Radar" O'Reilly could hear the choppers approaching before anyone else, and finish the sentences and read the minds of both of his commanding officers.

"Doctor Weinkle, don't you want to give this girl an MMR vaccine today?"

"Doesn't he also need an eye exam today?"

"You wanted me to call this patient to see if she's actually coming to her appointment, since she no-showed the last three times."

You know, Radar.

It's a running joke between us, but it's also proof of a deeper truth in medicine. As much as I've spent the last five chapters talking about a single relationship, that between the doctor and the patient, that relationship can't exist in a vacuum any longer. In the morass of modern healthcare, that relationship depends on dozens of other relationships, many of which don't directly involve the patient *or* the doctor, in order to survive.

The attentive resident learns about that interdependence early in training. Late one night in my second year of residency, a few days before a thankless Thanksgiving on call, I was pushing with the weight of my entire body on the femoral artery of an elderly woman, whose heroic stroke treatment had gone horribly awry. Instead of just busting the clot in her brain, the blood thinning medication had caused her to start leaking her whole blood volume out through the large hole punctured in her groin for the purpose of delivering the meds where they needed to go. The pressure dressings had failed, as had the "sandbags," and now we—meaning me—were resorting to the old-fashioned method, direct manual pressure.

On another floor, someone else unknown to me was in equally bad, if not worse, shape, and my reliable attending was hunkered down there. Neither of us had a free, or clean, hand to use the phone. And I did not know what to do next.

But Allison did. Fifteen years a critical care nurse, but only three hours into working with me, she was sizing me up. "Want me to order some platelets, doc?" she asked.

Yes. I most certainly did. "Thanks, Allison, yes. She had a type and screen before the procedure." I hesitated—I was supposed to order something else to stop this mess.

"What about a dose of vitamin K? Some fresh frozen plasma?"

Of course! That's what I needed. "FFP—the K will take too long to work."

She was smiling—I was still forgetting something.

"Want me to get one of the techs to spell you there before your arm falls off?"

Healing People, Not Patients

Oh right, that's what I was forgetting—I couldn't feel my fingers anymore, and I had eight other patients needing semi-urgent attention. Jeff, the nurse's aide, slid in beside me, and we counted three together, then replaced my hands with his. I stripped off the sticky, bloody gloves I was wearing, washed myself raw up to my elbows, and turned to grab my coat and go. Allison was already halfway through yelling at the blood bank to step on it by the time I cleared the automatic doors.

About 6 the next morning, I passed back through the same section of the ICU to check on the lady, whose bleeding had stopped quite nicely—and just as importantly, was moving all her limbs on her own. Allison was at the desk, feet propped on the next chair, dictating report and drinking coffee.

"You really kept your cool last night, doc," she complimented me. In 15 years, she had seen lots of screaming, out-of-control residents.

"That's only because you saved my butt," I replied.

ICU care, when it's done well, has been likened to a pit crew. Everyone has a spot that they stand in, a job that they do, and a single unified purpose they are pursuing. One person is in charge—but that person is dependent on everyone else's feedback, and when one of them sees a problem or makes a suggestion, even the team leader has to stop, integrate that feedback into the plan, and make sure the plan is still appropriate. It epitomizes the calm in the eye of the storm.

The rest of the healthcare system? Less of a pit crew, more like just the pits.

Every player on the team brings something critical to the table, possibly even something life-saving. The medical student makes the diagnosis of Graves' disease that eluded the attending. The patient confides in the social worker that she is being beaten regularly by her husband, which the doctor has suspected for years, but which the patient has always denied. The medical assistant gets the insurance to approve the crucial medication that finally gives the patient long-awaited relief.

It stands to reason, then, that every player on the team can make critical mistakes that will ruin the relationship just as easily. The critical question is whether our attitude is that we have each other's backs, or that we will readily throw each other under the bus. On the one hand, I remember one Sunday morning in residency, when I was taken to task by an attending over a note I had written as a favor to a classmate who needed help wrapping up with his patients so he could leave on time. I was never directly responsible for the child's care, but when the attending spotted a minor inaccuracy in the note, she called me immediately, very upset. "It doesn't matter that you were only responsible for this child for one hour," she fumed. "Once you assume *any* responsibility, you assume full responsibility."

I remember other nights in residency, in the very same hospital, being told to "batch my calls" with other residents before contacting the attending. The message was clearly that I needed to handle things myself, a virtual "do-not-disturb" sign. The extreme example of this was a story I was told while I was still a student by my chairman of medicine about his own intern year. On his very first day on service he admitted a patient with an unstable GI bleed. As evening approached, one of the nurses asked the attending what to do overnight. The attending smiled, indicated the intern who would become my chair, and said, "I'm sure this very capable intern can handle it."

Four years later, I was struggling with the ICU fellow to transfer a patient in myxedema coma, a life-threatening complication of thyroid disease, as he suggested I could probably handle things on the regular floor. I remembered and quoted my chairman's reply, "I cannot handle it, and the fact that I am telling you I lack the knowledge and resources to handle this makes it your responsibility to come down here and help me."

That shared responsibility can't just exist in the high-pressure environments of the hospital wards and critical care units; it needs to start at the front door of the primary care office and the back corridors of radiology.

Sometimes, the best teacher to a physician is the experiences he has as a patient. About 11 years ago, I had the monumental bad luck (and lack of coordination) to trip and fall on a concrete floor, while attending the wedding of a residency classmate in New Jersey. I fractured my left patella and cut my chin badly enough to need stitches, and ended up at 3 a.m. in the nearly deserted emergency room of a hospital in the shadow of Giants' Stadium.

On my way for x-rays, the transporter, clearly bored, gave my wheelchair a casual shove *and let go*, allowing me to roll unrestrained about halfway down the hallway, my injured leg sticking straight out, so it would be the first thing to crash into a wall. I was too shocked to say anything to him, but I was so angry that from that point on, I was looking for reasons to be dissatisfied. The flippant way the doctor told me about the x-ray findings ("Well, three of the bones in your knee are fine!"), his slipshod exam (I had a chin laceration, and he never checked whether my sore jaw was in alignment, a standard exam that I knew he should have done), and his disregard for hygiene (I needed to remind him to remove his gloves and wash before he began stitching my chin, since I had been watching him like a hawk since he came in the room, and he never approached the sink) did not go unnoticed. The transporter had destroyed any chance I had for a positive experience in the hospital, and when the inevitable "patient satisfaction survey" came in the mail a month later I eviscerated both him and the doctor, detailing my extreme *dis*-satisfaction.

Rarely is the gaffe this obvious. Often, the negative interactions are subtle enough that a reasonable bystander wouldn't necessarily find fault with anyone, but the damage still occurs. My colleague David, a doc in another primary care practice, found his patient Mrs. Kass not seated in the usual chair, but pacing furiously in the room.

"Oh doctor, thank God you're here. You must do something about that horrible woman out front who checked me in!" David froze. He had professional, dedicated front office staff. Indeed, they were among the things he treasured most in this job, and hearing any of them referred to so negatively got his hackles up.

"Who—I mean which—what happened, exactly?" He was caught off guard enough that he couldn't really decide what he wanted to know—and what he didn't.

Mrs. Kass waved a small index card in his face, too close and too rapidly for David to actually see anything. "She thinks I'm either crazy or a liar! 2:15! That's what this card that she gave me said, and here she's trying to tell me I'm late, and can't be seen!"

"But, you're—" David began, but didn't get any farther than that.

"In a room, yes, well no thanks to her. I grabbed someone who actually looked like they knew what they were doing, and she at least put me in a room, though not without making excuses for the idiot out front. I certainly hope you'll put a stop to it. I will NOT put up with this again, no matter how good of a doctor you are!"

David was in a bind. He had a solid working relationship with his front office—in fact, he treasured them, among other reasons because they "protected" him from late-arriving patients. This usually worked well when the patient acknowledged the lateness—in this case, however, there was a disagreement, and something didn't go well in the conduct of the disagreement, and now Mrs. Kass was angry at everyone. This was especially unfortunate, because despite her short temper, David had a good relationship with Mrs. Kass as well, having overcome a lot of her suspicion of doctors over the years and reached a good therapeutic alliance—which was now in serious jeopardy. Should he have thrown the front office under the bus to preserve his relationship with the patient? Or, was he such a team player that he would defend his staff as consummate professionals, even if it cost him his connection with Mrs. Kass?

Another colleague, Gabriela, works in a surgical subspecialty, and most of her patients have potentially life-threatening illnesses. She has seen her share of Mrs. Kasses in her career. Not long ago, she was interviewing a new nurse. "Look," she said to one candidate, "these people are at wits' end, really stressed out. They may say things or make requests that are absolutely ridiculous—and you need to roll with that. They will share with us all kinds of things, and we can really help them, but if we start out by pushing back, *they will shut down*. From that point on, they will have plenty to say—all of it nasty things about us." Gabriela paused at this point in her story, but I knew what was coming next. "If that doesn't sound like something you can handle, then this probably isn't the right job for you."

Part of the problem in making amends with patients like Mrs. Kass, when things go wrong, isn't the fault of the attitudes of the employees, though—it's the fact that priorities in healthcare are often muddled. It sometimes seems like the priority of caring for the patient is placed in conflict with some other supposed priority: protecting the doctor's time, preventing someone from accidentally getting medicine that the insurance won't pay for, getting "important" paperwork completed before a test is run, or adhering slavishly to a schedule, whether it be a chemotherapy protocol or an appointment schedule.

Doctors and administrators are given the privilege of deciding which priority holds sway. People at other levels of the hierarchy, however, often lack clear guidance as to what the most important priority. To further impede the patient from getting what they need, access to the doctor or administrator is often restricted—even for the other employees. A closed exam room door or a gowned, gloved surgeon in the OR means that everything else needs to wait—permissions, signatures, answers to pressing questions. The rest of the staff isn't empowered to make those decisions or help the patient.

My partner has a running joke about a limo driver who once advised her not to argue with people. "Just do what I do when someone asks me to go the wrong way down a one-way street—say, 'Lemme see what I can do for you.'" While I'm not advocating flouting the traffic laws in Manhattan (or anywhere else), the limo driver is on to something. The power of "Lemme see what I can do for you" is that we are on the same team, trying to solve a problem together. I would love to hear "Lemme see what I can do for you" become the default response, instead of just, "No."

I would have especially loved it when I was working on getting Teresa's sleep study approved. Teresa, who is in her mid-60s and has had sleep apnea for 15 years, realized her equipment had finally worn out. The insurer had been paying regularly for maintenance of the equipment, but now that it was no longer functional, the representative insisted they would need a new sleep study to approve new equipment, in case the patient's disease had worsened over the years. They did not, however, specify which of the two commonly ordered sleep studies would be needed. We ordered the one we thought was appropriate—and guessed incorrectly. The second representative rejected the order and told the nurse I needed to call a "peer reviewer," meaning a physician working for the insurance company, to discuss the case.

These reviews are a massive inconvenience. The reviewers work bankers' hours and are always away from their desks or on another call when I do get free to call them. I am forced to leave a call-back time, which is only my vain hope of when I am praying to be free to speak with them. Whenever I can, I try to find an alternative way to resolve the problem. In this case, I tried to simply cancel my original order, since it was an honest mistake attributable to poor instructions, and submit a new, correct order.

What happened next defied all logic. "You can't cancel the order now," representative #2 told us. "You have to go through the peer review, let them reject the order, and *then* you can cancel it and order the correct study." I had no choice but to play phone tag with the reviewing physician—for the sole purpose of being told no, so I could do what common sense would dictate I should do all along.

Healing People, Not Patients

Finally, after far too much time had gone by, I made contact with the dismayed reviewer. As I explained the entire sequence of events to her, I could swear I heard her rhythmically banging her head on her desk. "I don't know why any of this happened," she apologized. "That rep should have approved the original study, based on the fact that she already uses the machine, and in fact she should have *both* studies done to figure out how bad the disease is and *then* decide what equipment to use and on what settings."

"I'm sorry you wasted so much time on this."

That crunching sound you heard was representative #2 being thrown under a bus by the physician reviewer. Lack of respect among members of the healthcare system is nearly as big a problem as disrespect shown directly to patients. It can percolate down through the system, so that a disrespected employee or trainee has no outlet for his frustration except to pass it along to the patients.

My medical school has a standing award, given by the graduating class, called the *Anus Equinus* (*equinus* = horse, *anus*—well, you know what that means). To earn the award, attendings and residents had done such egregious things as head-butting a student across the operating table if they answered a question incorrectly. My own nominee for the award once told me, when I informed her that I would be missing a day for the beginning of Passover, "It's more work for me when you're here anyway." Later that month, however, she was incredulous to find that I had not come to work the Monday after my first son was born—while my wife was still hospitalized. Yet, this same resident won an award *in that same year* for her meticulous attention to legible notes and clear communication in the chart. Guess my dignity was less important than neat handwriting.

My experience with the sleep study closely resembles what happens to a lot of my patients, especially the ones who have limited English, when they go to the pharmacy to pick up medications. Still unfamiliar with the US system of prescription pharmacies, they come to me and say, "That medication is finished now. I went to the pharmacy to get it, and they say I cannot have it." Rather than contact me, the pharmacy simply turns the patient away, without medication and without an explanation of how to fix the problem. They are preferring efficiency over courtesy—keeping the pharmacy line moving, rather than addressing the patient's immediate need.

I used to think the problem was one of empathy: the pharmacist's idea of what is inconvenient is different from the patient's, because they have different priorities. Since the pharmacist suffers no adverse consequence for the patient's inconvenience of not getting the prescription, there is no intrinsic motivation to solve the problem, but a strong motivation (time pressure) to say, "I can't help you," and move on. Only when the person providing the service can empathize with the patient need, to get the medicine because the next time they will be able to speak to the physician will not be for three months, is there a chance of overriding the pharmacist's priorities to help the patient.

I now realize that it isn't always empathy that's lacking—it's agency, the belief that the pharmacy employee actually has the power to do something for the patient. Just like there are different cultures of how residents do or do not look out for each other, each pharmacy has its own culture. I've had experiences where two different pharmacies in the same chain behaved as though they were on different planets. One routinely sends my patients who don't speak English away without medication or explanation. The other, located maybe five miles away, employs a pharmacist who once called me because she was worried about a particular patient, spent 20 minutes on the phone with me comparing medication lists, informed me that the patient had an English-speaking neighbor who often came in to pick up meds for her, *and provided me with that neighbor's number.* She recognized what I had been taught, the hard way, that bleary-eyed Sunday in residency—all of us are responsible for the patient's well-being, even if we only touch their lives for 10 seconds, even if we never lay eyes on the patient (and many pharmacists don't, since the technicians are usually the ones staffing the pickup window).

People like this pharmacist, or our front office staff, or the café worker who makes the sandwiches at the hospital where I do newborn rounds, remind me of a story I once heard from Richard Joel, at the time the president of Hillel International and now the president of Yeshiva University:

A reporter was roaming the grounds of Mount Moriah as Solomon's Temple was being built, trying to score a big story for the next day's edition of the *Times of Ancient Israel.*

"What do you do here?" the reporter asked a laborer who was dragging a sledge with heavy stone blocks on it.

"Why, I transport the bricks," said the laborer.

"Thank you very much," said the reporter, and moved on to the next site, where a second laborer was banging a hammer on a sheet of bronze.

"What do you do?" asked the reporter, hoping for a juicier answer this time.

"Oh, my job is very important—I'm a skilled craftsman, and I am making the bronze laver. Now, if you'll excuse me, I am way behind schedule."

Better, thought the reporter, but something was still missing. He came upon a third laborer who was vigorously sweeping up with a broom.

The janitor harrumphed the reporter, but the day was growing long, so he tried his hand.

"What do you do," he asked the janitor.

The janitor stopped his sweeping, held his broom upright and beamed. "I am building the Temple to the Glory of God Almighty."

People who can be like that janitor, keeping their eyes on the prize, on the whole picture, even while doing mundane or repetitive tasks, keep the whole system going. They are more likely to look out for situations in which the patient's needs are being overshadowed by something else in the system.

Like when patients wait. At. The. Doctor's. Office. For. *Ever.*

The covenant we make with patients is that their needs are going to become as important to us as our own. Their lives are as dear as our lives. We are as careful about spending their money for them, as we would be with our own. And if the old sayings are true—"Time is money;" "living on borrowed time;" "don't want to waste any more of your valuable time"—then their time should be as precious as our own.

Instead, wasted time at the doctor's office is so common, so expected, that my patients routinely plan to take the entire day off from work for their doctor's appointments. Every doctor I know has had patients threaten to charge them for their time spent waiting, the way lawyers bill in six-minute intervals. One patient advocate, Laura Casey, grew so exasperated with waits in the doctor's office that she coined a new phrase for them: "lost lifetime." Ouch.

My late grandfather and I got our medical care from the same internal medicine practice, but from different doctors. When I was helping to guide him through his difficult decisions near the end of his life, I accompanied him to a visit with his PCP. In the waiting room, I noticed a new feature to the office I hadn't seen before: a white board. On the board were the names of all the doctors seeing patients in the office that day, followed by one piece of information: how many minutes behind schedule they were. In particular, I noticed two names: my grandfather's doctor, listed as 45 minutes behind, and my own, listed as "on time." He was the only one.

Another legendary internist in my hometown has trained generations of medical students in the examination of the thyroid and the art of thinking through a problem before ordering a bunch of tests. Students love his lectures, delivered without notes and packed full of clinical anecdotes to illustrate a point. Yet, I've talked to many who assiduously avoided being placed with him for a clinical rotation, because this master physician would habitually finish clinic somewhere around midnight—and the diminutive elderly Italian and Polish immigrant women who made up the bulk of his patients would wait right until the end, steadfastly sticking by their doctor who always did right by them. The legendary master had built a trust with these women by never glancing at his watch or the clock, never standing to speak with them, when he could sit instead, never rushing them through a visit, that when it was their turn, they would have his undivided attention for as long as it took.

It's not that I've interviewed these women to find this out; my own practice teaches me this lesson. The other day I had to call and apologize to a mother of one of my patients who had brought her daughter in on time, gotten checked in, roomed, and even spoken for a while with the medical student. While all of that was happening, I was seeing another older man who needed far more time than the 15 minutes allotted, and his daughter who had been squeezed into my schedule as an urgent visit after three trips to the ER.

By the time I was done, it was about an hour past the first girl's visit time. I girded myself for a groveling apology, opened the door to the room—and found it empty. When I called the mother from my desk a few minutes later, however, she was sweet as could be. "No, I completely understand. You're busy and needed to make sure you did a good job with the previous patients. You always spend plenty of time with us when we need it—we'll reschedule and come back soon. Thanks for everything you've done."

Think of it like waiting in a restaurant. If you're in line for cheap, fast food, and you find yourself waiting more than about five minutes, you are not going to be pleased. If you are waiting in a candlelit dining room for a "slow food" meal in a tiny town hanging off the side of a seaside hill in Southern Italy, you could sit for an hour between courses and not notice the time passing. If the time you get to spend with your clinician is unhurried, satisfying, and purposeful, then there is every reason to lean back with a good book and wait your turn. If the clinician blows through the door, never looks up from his notes, and rushes back out again five minutes later, you will be angry at having waited two hours for *that*.

Likewise, the rest of the system can make the wait worthwhile, or worthless, depending on how it's handled. I've called colleagues at their offices, and the receptionist answers, "Experts in Internal Medicine, can you hold please?" and before I can even say, "Actually, no, I can't hold," I am on hold. And that's when I call the "private back line" for clinicians. Imagine what my patients are going through—they are waiting, before they even get to say hello, let along learn that their doctor is doing an extended hand-holding session with the previous patient.

There are delays and redundancies at every stage of the process. I've done some training in quality improvement that incorporates techniques from the industrial process world—Toyota Production System, Six Sigma, LEAN, whichever label you want to put on it. The process to get someone's blood drawn and labeled for the lab, the system for making a new appointment, or the path someone walks to get from the front desk to the exam room can all look like a mass of tangled spaghetti, or like the old Family Circus cartoons, in which Billy comes home from the neighbor's house by way of the dump, the playground, and a construction site. At each stage, the patient sits and waits in a chair, with no notification of what they're waiting for, how long they'll be there, or who it was that put them there.

It's not easy to fix this; a practice can struggle for literally years trying to streamline and staff the phone system. A fully staffed front desk can improve access—until there is employee turnover, whether due to staff seeking other jobs, or being reassigned by a parent health system. Adding providers and nurses can shorten response times to patient calls and requests for appointments—but possibly at the expense of continuity, because more of those calls and appointments will involve a nurse or provider who is essentially a stranger to that patient. We run into this in my own practice, despite our concerted efforts to maintain "empanelment," but we must be doing comparatively well, because time and again, I get new patients transferring in because "at my old doctor's office, I never saw the same person two times in a row."

The waiting and shuffling around can make a patient feel devalued and depersonalized—they stop being their own person with their own doctor and become a generic patient who can see a generic doctor or speak to a generic nurse. It is hard to know where the tipping point is between feeling devalued because you feel like a stranger, and feeling devalued because someone is wasting your time—but even worse when you end up feeling like you got neither speedy service nor personal attention.

There's a new movement afoot in primary care that is supposed to address this problem, called the medical home concept. I always think of a medical home as a return to the "good old days," when most doctors were solo practitioners who did everything, and a patient, especially in a smaller town, could expect care that *felt* like home. A familiar face. Care that actually took place in their home, or in the doctor's home (in a converted carriage house or separate entrance used as an office). Continuity throughout their life, delivering the babies, casting the 10-year-old's broken arm, treating the flu, managing the blood pressure, and accompanying them through old age. Presence wherever and whenever it was needed, in the middle of the night, meeting them in the emergency room or coming to round in the hospital, the nursery, or in a neighbor's yard after a nasty fall.

Neither society nor the medical system works like this anymore. There are too many different kinds of care, too many locations where it takes place, and too many demands on a doctor's time to enable this kind of practice in all but the smallest and most remote of towns. Hospital privileges, insurance credentialing, and the simple fact that doctors have belatedly learned that we can't work 168-hour weeks and maintain our own health and family relationships prevent us from being like our favorite docs of yesteryear.

The medical home model is trying to meet a more modest goal. With all of the fragmentation and discontinuity, the medical system is the proverbial five blind men examining an elephant. No one has any idea of the big picture, because each is only examining one small part of the patient, or one snapshot of the patient in time. The emergency physician only sees what is happening at 11 p.m. on Wednesday, because his only job is to stabilize the patient at 11 p.m. on Wednesday. The cardiologist only looks at what's inside that little box in the middle of the chest, like in the story I told in Chapter 1. Someone needs to know the whole patient, something that most of my *patients* struggle to do, if their medical histories are complex enough.

The problem with the medical home model is that it can end up being the kind of home described by Robert Frost in "Death of the Hired Man:" "When you have to go there, they have to take you in." The process of becoming a medical home is tedious, detailed, and based on meeting a lot of population metrics that involve doing the same thing every time for every person in the practice who fits a certain category—screening tests for depression, blood sugar testing in diabetics, completing the full panel of vaccines in all children by age two. Patients with complicated life situations can throw a major monkey wrench into the process, and medical home interactions can easily devolve into haranguing them so the practice can check off the box: "Mr. Cartwright, I know it's really hard to catch the bus, but we need to make sure you come in and get your blood pressure measured before the end of the month."

I'm more interested in a proactive version of the medical home. Several years ago, a mother of four girls in my practice turned to me and said, "You know, we always have a hard time remembering to schedule the girls' visits and get them their shots—I really want a practice where we're getting reminders of when those things are supposed to happen." She was looking for the kind of "home" where, if you didn't show up for dinner on time, someone went out looking for you. It's as a different writer, the medieval poet Judah HaLevi described it: "And in my going out to meet you, I found you coming toward me."

Not just coming toward me to remind me to take my medicine, either. Coming toward me to find out how I'm doing, because I haven't been in for a long time. Coming toward me to see if the new medication I just started is working, useless, or making my hair fall out and my tongue turn green. Coming toward me because I've been in the emergency room 20 times this year, and people care enough to worry if I am addicted to drugs, severely ill without a clear diagnosis—or homeless and seeking convenient shelter.

Getting routine care and timely disease-specific treatment is hugely important—but so is just knowing that the doctor and nurses and everyone else is worried about me. My depressed patients often describe passive death wishes that center around the rumination that, "No one would miss me if I died." The least we can do as healers is demonstrate convincingly that *we* would miss them, even before they ask.

Really doing this well takes more than a medical home—it takes a medical community, a medical neighborhood, if you will. Any medical home project that happens solely under one roof these days is doomed to fail. Primary care doctors need relationships, real person-talking-to-other-person relationships, with specialists, hospitalists, and emergency rooms. Doctors and nurses need to get to know pharmacists on a first name basis, have phone conversations with physical therapists, e-mail school nurses and teachers, and build alliances with community organizations, home-care agencies, and advocacy groups. Emergency rooms need to think outside their walls

Healing People, Not Patients

and engage in issues of gun violence, lack of follow-up, and housing instability—like the "hotspotting" initiatives in Camden, New Jersey.

In Pittsburgh, there is a "community paramedic" program that I learned about when one of my patients, who was a "frequent flier" in several local ERs, came to a visit accompanied by an EMT. This paramedic said she had been assigned to help keep Patty out of the emergency room by reminding her, to fill meds and reviewing her symptoms with her so she didn't panic when she felt something was wrong.

The medical home I work in embraces this approach. Sure, we still keep track of blood sugars and of how many people have gotten their pneumonia vaccines. But, we do a lot of coming towards our patients as well. We've worked with nearby schools to strengthen their vaccine requirements for school entry, so we don't become the next focus of a preventable disease outbreak. We've built relationships with the refugee resettlement agencies that refer so many of our new patients to us, so that we can actually make an impact on the "non-medical" issues that are the real source of so many illnesses we try to treat. We've made contacts in school offices around the area, the Epilepsy Foundation, the mental health agencies, and the health department, so that we can provide extra support for adult and pediatric patients with chronic illnesses. And since 2010, we've brought the mobile unit (remember the Winnebago?) to a half-dozen different community agencies to bring on-site medical care to patients who would have trouble coming to us.

On a personal level, I've taken a cue from my medical assistant and learned to anticipate needs. New immigrants and teenagers need driver's physicals. Three-year-olds need vaccine records for pre-school. Elderly immigrants whom I've been seeing for five years will need to have their memory tested to see if they can take the citizenship exam (thank you, Kee May). And chronically ill people who have trouble getting themselves dressed and making their meals will need forms for Social Security and certification for in-home caregiving. I've filled my Dropbox with blank copies of every imaginable form and saved e-mail contacts for people from every conceivable agency.

It doesn't seem like enough. In an ideal world, I'd find a way to keep in touch with everyone I take care of—but I have enough trouble keeping tabs on my close friends and family, and I have literally a few thousand patients. I am bound to miss something. I need some method—a "worry list," a daily report reminding me I haven't seen or heard from someone in six months, or just a swift kick in the pants—of moving myself to check up on the people who need to hear from me.

There's a lot of inertia to overcome. The tendency to think that "no news is good news" or "out of sight, out of mind" lulls me, as well as many of my colleagues, into thinking that everything must be fine, or we would have heard something. In reality, however, there's a lot of emergency rooms out there, a lot of other providers, and a lot of people who simply suffer in silence and don't seek care when they should. This is what the poet meant; by the time the patient decides they need to come seeking me, I should already be coming toward them, seeking them out, wondering how they are doing.

I think of Harriet, the woman who got so upset about her mammogram prescription, even though she had told me already she knew she was dying. I planned several trips to visit her in hospice, and delayed each. I had finally cleared my schedule for Thursday afternoon to head over there, until the phone rang at 11 a.m. Thursday. It was her husband; she had died an hour before. I need to get better at this.

Lately, I've noticed that my practice is trying to create the same tone among employees, as well. I came back from a long vacation last month and found two weeks' worth of mail sitting on my desk—divided into neat, labeled piles by a proactive nurse. A board has gone up in the lunchroom with photos and personal vignettes about staff members in every role, four people each month, corresponding with the anniversary of when they started work. Staff members remind each other to eat, volunteer their lunches to each other when someone forgets, organize soup swaps, and routinely check in with each other when someone seems to be having a bad mental health day. Just like the malignant attitudes of supervisors and superiors I mentioned earlier can percolate down the hierarchy, so can positive ones like this. A quart of good homemade soup buys a lot of good will.

So does homemade chocolate or a crayon drawing of a butterfly. These aren't items I've gotten from co-workers, but from patients and their children. I keep the butterfly, and a lot of other patient artwork and thank you notes on my desk, partially as a reminder that we can't build the medical home or the health community from one side of the relationship alone. There have to be *mutual* obligations, otherwise this relationship isn't a covenant—it is that thing that the modern healthcare *industry* keeps pushing, namely a consumer relationship, where the "service provider" has all the responsibility and the consumer has none.

Our services can be bought, then discarded for those of another person who is cheaper, faster, or closer to home. For those of us in the healthcare professions who feel like it is our calling in life to heal, finding our profession becoming an exercise in retail sales is a sure recipe for burnout. While retail clinics may serve a purpose in a pinch, the covenant between patient and doctor is what takes us over the line from fixing to healing, from health maintenance to well-being. Maintaining that relationship takes input from the patient, as well as from the medical system.

The most important obligation the patient has is actually to view themselves as a valuable human being. A patient shouldn't feel they need to apologize for taking up "the doctor's valuable time"—what better to occupy the doctor's valuable time than another human being's valuable life and the problems they are encountering in that life. Beyond simple self-esteem, however, every physician I know would ask the patient to *behave* as though they value that life—engaging in healthy, life-enriching behaviors when well, making a good-faith effort to heal when ill, and working as an active partner with the healer to live as well as they can at that moment. We like activated patients—people who walk into our office determined to get better and stay that way, and walk out and actually do something about it.

Healing People, Not Patients

Activated patients read—they read what their doctors tell them to read, what their friends tell them to read, and they go out looking in libraries and online for information. They take a diagnosis as an imperative to become an expert on that diagnosis, a prescription as an invitation to research the side effects of the medicines, and a setback in treatment as an opportunity to learn about all the alternatives. Activated patients also take action—they dive headlong into rehabilitation programs, attend support groups, journal their experiences, and communicate with their healers by email or web portals. And activated patients ask questions—to challenge, to clarify, and to anticipate.

Activated patients also scare a lot of healers. A lot of us dread going to work the morning after a *Grey's Anatomy* episode airs, hope for TV talk-show doctors to all be simultaneously struck with a plague of laryngitis, and pray for the WebMD site to crash—permanently. Mass media can have the effect of devaluing the expertise that we bring to the table for patients we know personally, and replacing it with a habit of demanding whatever is trending. And replacing *us*, too, if we don't step to it and produce the service right away. Designer lab tests, expensive supplements, just-released "me-too" medications, and referrals to "the national expert in my condition" all pressure us to give the patient what they want or risk our valued relationship.

I don't believe in the idea of "following the doctor's orders," as if I am a military commander. I don't even like using the similarly passive, subservient word "compliant" to describe whether someone is taking their medications. Doctors need a healthy amount of humility, in order to recognize that we don't know everything, and even if we know more than the patient, they know themselves better than we do most of the time.

On the other hand, patients need enough humility to acknowledge that they came to us because they had a problem they could not solve alone, one we trained for a decade to be able to address. I mean the kind of humility that enables them to listen in earnest to the advice I provide, and bringing information from outside not in order to be confrontational or dismissive, but in order to foster discussion and reach the common goal of the patient's wellness. We're like people studying a text together, with criticism and commentary—the text is the patient's body and illness, and the commentaries are the TV shows, the latest edition of MedPage Today, and the last Internet ad to "talk to your doctor about your poop."

Valuing our expertise is only part of the equation, though. I just talked about how the system needs to value the patient's time; in a healthy relationship that respect is reciprocated. Sure, a lot of wasted time is due to inefficiency and a general lack of pro-active behavior in the healthcare system. But, some of the wait for an appointment is caused by people who will not show up for their already booked appointments. Some of the wait in the waiting room is caused by overbooking to compensate for the anticipated no-shows, or because the healer and the patient wasted an appointment discussing why the patient has not yet called the specialist to whom they were referred several appointments ago, or taken the medicine that was recommended as highly effective treatment over a year ago. A patient who doesn't value the provider's time also ends up wasting the time of *other patients.* Doctors don't exist in a vacuum—turns out patients don't either.

Patients also need to be able to place their trust in us. That's hard to do; many of the patients I care for have long personal histories of having their trust betrayed, sometimes by doctors, other times by governments, friends, family, or a combination of everyone they've ever known. They are many times bitten and always shy, and will never trust or share easily.

Physicians and other healthcare professionals, on the other hand, are steeped in a culture of confidentiality that long predates the HIPAA legislation of the past two decades. The reason for this confidentiality is simple: the symptoms, signs, causes and consequences of illness, and even the circumstances of wellness, in a person's life are delicate, embarrassing, or even shocking. Confidence in, well, confidence is the only way for most people to be reassured enough that they can unload on the healer, without fear that the story will find its way onto the front page of the newspaper, into the ear of the village gossip, or back to a suspicious spouse or parent—or be used by the provider in some way to hurt or take advantage of them. Protecting the confidentiality of minors so that they can open up to a tight-lipped physician about sexuality, drug use, and other "risk-taking" behavior is one of the key elements in addressing those behaviors and treating their after-effects, before irreparable harm comes to the adolescent.

However, all of that confidentiality is far less useful if a patient won't use it to share the full story. I can listen attentively, ask all the right questions, and say all the right things, but if the narrative is left deliberately unfinished, how can I be sure of reading it correctly? If you don't tell me about the torture you endured before you fled your country, I can't make the case that your terrible anxiety disorder is actually post-traumatic stress that qualifies you for asylum. If you didn't mention the horrible argument with your first husband that happened just before he died of a heart attack, I can make much less sense of the terrible chest pain you get whenever there is conflict in your current relationship. A patient can count on me to guard their secrets with my life—but if they guard their secrets from me, that often makes it much more difficult for me to guard their life.

Far more often, I encounter patients who withhold more pedestrian secrets. They are still coughing not because my stupid medicines don't work, but because they were too embarrassed to tell me they had resumed smoking. The seizure they had in the hospital was not a surprise to them, even though it scared the living daylights out of the nurses, because they have had epilepsy since childhood, but didn't tell me, because their parents told them it was something to be ashamed of. They didn't mention the blood in their stool for the last six months, because they didn't think it was important enough to bring up. And of course, the untold stories of erectile dysfunction, depression, anxiety, bowel and bladder dysfunction, and, in bygone days, even breast cancer that were kept quiet due to stigma and stereotype. When the information comes out, the physician feels much like a person whose spouse forgot to pass on an important message: "Well, that would have been helpful to know!"

Forthrightness doesn't end with the patient's own dirty laundry and unpleasant symptoms, though. Just like I need to find ways to tactfully rebuke a patient sometimes, the patient needs to do the same to me, on occasion. A medicine did not work as planned, or had unpleasant side effects or even a frightening allergic reaction. The anticipated quick recovery never came, and the disease got much worse and ended the patient up in the hospital. The prescription was never sent to the pharmacy. I must be able to receive criticism as well as deliver it; the patient who encounters a problem needs to be willing to share it, rather than silently disappearing from my practice, or serving me with a lawsuit, even though the problem may have arisen despite a good faith effort to achieve healing. I need to be cautious with my patients—not afraid of them.

Of course, each of these obligations assumes that all of us in the medical home have done our part. I can't expect a patient to bare their soul—or their body—if the door is left open, the questions are asked in a sneering manner, or the nurse's body language suggests that they are completing a form, rather than helping to heal. I can't assume that a patient has "blown off" an appointment without calling to ensure that they are well, determining if their car broke down or their bus didn't come, or discovering that they are afraid to come in because their insurance termed, and they didn't think I would see them anymore. Furthermore, I can't label a patient "difficult," because they tell me that doctors don't know what they're talking about, but Doctor Oz does, when it becomes clear that they tried casually raising questions they had after doing Internet research with three other doctors before you, only to have all of the doctors tell them that they should quit looking stuff up. A true mutual relationship doesn't involve each party going in 50 percent—it involves each party striving to go the distance—and being pleasantly surprised to find the other meeting him halfway.

empathy

health duty

touch lifestyle illness physician honor

rapport courtesy

experience listening covenant

disorder communication faith

drugs dignity life feeling hearing

death healthcare people medicine non-verbal therapy exercise

respect

share relationships nurse collaborate sickness

healing understanding nutrition

wellness treatment humanity

pain cure

patients

disease

healer

compassion

bond

CHAPTER 7

Strangers

"When you are a refugee, you are nowhere."

Well-spoken, well-dressed, declining the translator, this man scarcely looked like someone scarcely three weeks in the US and barely over his jet lag. He looked even less like someone who had just arrived from the very fringes of human existence.

"Doctor, my wife fell ill, she and the child. But, in our place, in the camp, there was no help, no medicine. Three weeks they were sick, and then they died. I am telling you this so you may understand; I do not know what was wrong with them. I am a refugee, I do not belong, and so, when they fall sick, I am nowhere. That is what it is like when you are a refugee—you are nowhere."

The news tells me that 60 million people in the world today are nowhere. Homeless, stateless, and often hopeless. Strangers in a strange land, to borrow an oft-borrowed phrase.

The shame of it is that when you are nowhere, it is hard to get decent medical care. Or any medical care. We can talk about seeing the humanity in each patient—but it's hard to see the humanity in someone whom you can't see at all, who isn't even on your radar. Purna, the lonely but dapper man before me, found himself off the medical grid at the very moment he most needed someone to recognize his, and his family's, humanity, and now he alone was escaped to tell me.

Around the same time, I met Tun, a Burmese-speaking man of few words and two fewer fingers than most. As I delved with him into the backache that always bothered him, I tried to probe for answers as to where the missing digits had gone. For all the progress I made, Tun might as well have just told me, "What missing fingers?" I learned even less of his time in Burma and what it was that made him flee one night across the border from the frying pan of Burma to the fire of Malaysia—where refugees live in hiding, in fear of police and informers who threaten to rob, beat, or deport them, even as they man the restaurants, auto body shops, and laundries of Kuala Lumpur. A couple words about forced labor and carrying heavy bags for the army, the same story I got from everyone.

This time, though, I had a student with me, herself of Burmese background and doubling as our translator. He was no more forthcoming with her than with me, but after Tun went home, she turned to me and said, "I think he's Rohingya."

We went back to my desk, and she gave me a crash tutorial on what it meant to be Rohingya. The term itself was probably meant to be derogatory, and was the Burmese label for Burmese-speaking Muslims living in the western part of the country. They have lived in their homes in Burma for generations, but the local non-Muslim population considers them illegal immigrants from Bangladesh. They are subjected to mob violence and have been forced from their homes in the hundreds of thousands, in a classic case of ethnic cleansing. They reside in refugee camps, cut off from many

Healing People, Not Patients

basic needs, including adequate healthcare for such issues as pregnancy. At some point a few years ago, several thousand of them ended up adrift in boats along the Malaysian coast, unwelcome either in Burma or in Malaysia. And most tragically, they have been led to believe, whether rightly or wrongly, that the medical system actually has it in for them, and that doctors from the majority group may harm or kill them, in order to keep them from seeking medical care. In a situation like that, I agreed, losing track of a couple fingers wouldn't be hard.

For Tun, coming to my attention may have been the first time in his life that he got medical care like a human being. It's easy to enthusiastically endorse the premise of this book that every person who comes to seek medical care deserves to be treated as a human being equal to those providing the care, or if you prefer, as a being created in God's image. It is easy to nod vigorously, when I repeat, "Love your neighbor as yourself." It is much harder to love someone who you can't see as your neighbor, whether it is because they couldn't afford to live in your neighborhood, wouldn't be allowed to live in your neighborhood, or would make your actual neighbors yell, "There goes the neighborhood," if they moved in next door. Strangeness can be so overwhelming, even to caring members of the healing professions, that it completely eclipses humanity.

How else to explain people who trained as physicians who were nevertheless able to participate in Mengele's twisted experiments in Auschwitz? How else to explain a series of American doctors, who over the course of *40 years*, kept their equanimity, while watching the African-American men who were the victims of the Tuskegee experiment grow sick and die of treatable syphilis? And how else to explain why people in Burma could simply decide that Tun and his fellow Rohingya didn't really deserve medical care? Whether we are blind to suffering or poisoned by prejudice, the healing arts can also inflict wounds just as easily as the rest of society, unless we learn to look beyond the strangeness to find the shared divinity in everyone.

Finding that shared humanity can be almost impossible, however, without the ability to communicate. I call the Arabic interpreter, only to find out that only one member of the Syrian family I'm talking to speaks Arabic—the rest speak Kurdish. But not regular Kurdish—Kurmanji. Oh, but not *that* dialect of Kurmanji—the other one. Then, halfway through the interview that I am finally conducting with the correct interpreter, I learn that the patient does not realize we are speaking about his health; he thinks this is a meeting with the doctor for him to tell me about his disabled brother for whom he is caring.

We're unusual, though; until recently only a few places, usually large academic hospitals on the coasts, offered interpretation services. So, I have had patients seen by other providers who "overcame" the language barrier by shouting louder. When I questioned how the patient could have understood them, their answer was, "Oh, she understood," even though I know full well her English is non-existent. One office manager even told our care manager, "You know, sometimes *they* pretend not to understand English, when *they* really do." Because pretending to be completely ignorant somehow benefitted them? I don't get it.

Even when interpretation services are available, they are not always used. I've arrived at a hospital at 7:00 in the morning to round on a patient admitted at 5:00 the previous afternoon only to discover that the double-handset "blue phone" still hasn't been delivered to their room. For the past 14 hours, they have been communicating to the nurses by pointing, smiling sweetly, and shrugging. When I have referred that same patient to a specialist after hospital discharge, they waited several extra weeks for the appointment, until a live interpreter could be scheduled, then got sent home when, after waiting more than an hour, the interpreter failed to show up. The office had blue phones available—but only by advance request, so they cannot substitute a phone translator on the spur of the moment. Blue phones are more valuable than Times Square apartments on New Years, apparently, and only one person in the hospital, the AOD, has the super power of bestowing them on the nursing units that need them. Wouldn't want 4 Main to stockpile too many extra translation phones, would we?

And even when everything goes right, and there is a translator available who speaks the correct language, I'm now trying to build a meaningful covenant with a patient through an intermediary, a filter. That filter can separate out the noise from the signal—or it can trap the most vital information I need to make this relationship work, information about that person's Lifeworld.

See, I don't live in the real world. I'm a doctor; I live in the medical reality, with its own set of concepts, priorities, and protocols, and with its own language that doesn't make sense to anyone else. But, my patients don't live in the medical reality—they each live in a Lifeworld filled with trials and tribulations that mean everything to them and suck up every ounce of attention they have. Even with a simple sickness, like strep throat or a laceration of the pinky finger, the Lifeworld impacts the illness, and the illness alters the Lifeworld.

Lifeworld is all the bits of information we talked about in Chapters 2 and 3, the details that we need to listen for and ask about that turn the facts of disease into the narrative of an illness, that tell us about the patient we're going to care for, instead of the disease in the textbook. The more Lifeworld is addressed in the conversation, the more mutually agreeable the outcome is for both healer and patient. But, what can I do if the Lifeworld never makes it onto my radar?

When I'm lucky, I stumble on one of my truly great phone translators, the ones I know by name and voice. They will follow a verbatim translation with a veritable cultural Wikipedia of explanations of all the euphemisms, metaphors, and untranslatable words the patient has just used. One Somali interpreter once interrupted the translation to tell me how the patient's reluctance to speak about a particular issue stemmed from the fact that the Somali community is very small and close-knit, even across state lines, and she was certain she must be speaking to someone she knew. His cultural translation

Healing People, Not Patients

saved my relationship with this patient, with whom I have since built a deep level of trust. Another interpreter managed through exact, careful translations of the patient's own words, to convey to me that a woman who had never been to school was, in fact, describing her neurological disorder in almost textbook terms, including changes that she could not possibly have felt as symptoms.

Even more valued are the "flesh-and-blood" translators, as I call them—our crew of in-person Nepali translators, who not only know the language and culture of the patients, but the mind of the doctors. They have taught me about holidays, customs, interesting cultural beliefs like the idea that eating cold food or drinking cold water causes heartburn, the history of the expulsion of their community from Bhutan, and elements of the Nepali language. My phone translators all laugh when they hear me use the correct Nepali word for Betel nut, and my patients laugh when I tell them in Nepali to lie down. The translators also empower many of the patients, by stepping into the background when they see the patient attempt to answer for themselves in English, letting the patient use them more as a crutch than as a go-between.

On the other hand, it's a mixed bag. As such, I am at the mercy of the schedule and whether my favorite phone translators are already on a call or taking the day off. Professional translators often see themselves as extensions of the medical establishment; they are likely better educated than the patients they are interpreting for and may see themselves, perhaps in keeping with their culture of origin, as superior for having been more assimilated into the new culture. As a result, the translator may, themselves, devalue the religious or cultural material being provided by the patient. At other times, they may feel that they have a responsibility to the doctor to "keep the patient on topic." Still other times, they may feel that they have to make an interpretive translation into English, rather than preserving the sense of the words the patient is saying.

Every time I ask a one-sentence question, and there is an animated exchange lasting five minutes before the interpreter answers, I fear that either my question or the reply has been stripped of the original meaning and replaced with what the translator thought it should mean. On occasion, I need to hang up and start again, when I hear the voice of one of the handful of interpreters that I refuse to use, because of past experience with them being rude or condescending to patients or even putting words in my mouth that I did not say.

For patients who have no way of hearing me but through this conduit of the interpreter, the interpreter's words are the only representation of me that they have. I can be as attentive and kind as I want. If my words are translated harshly, however, that is all they will hear. One of the interpreters that I no longer use lost my confidence when he said, "She said this, but she is a very uneducated person, so she does not know the word that she means, so I am having to use a different word instead."

Sometimes, the blocking is even worse because of inherent conflicts between patient and interpreter. One Pakistani teenager demanded I hang up with his Urdu translator and either get a Hindi translator online or continue in his mediocre English.

After securing the Hindi translator, he revealed that something about the Urdu-speaking man's accent made him dead certain that the translator belonged to the tribe that had torched his village, and was lying to me about what was wrong with the patient's health. My Iraqi and Syrian patients will only discuss issues of reproduction and genitalia with a translator of their own gender—and occasionally won't even use the translator, so they either keep the information to themselves or struggle to explain it to me by drawing pictures and breaking their teeth on the English words. And my partner once had to discontinue a call because the patient revealed that he knew the phone interpreter's voice, because they had been in the refugee camp together.

Best practices for interpretation dictate that family members should *never* be used as medical translators. The family member, usually the younger, more educated member of the family, often has the same motivation as the professional to appear Westernized, or to keep the visit on topic. Often, the person translating has their own agenda: safety precautions for someone who is falling, or hiring a caregiver, or an exemption from taking the citizenship exam. These are time-consuming processes, which often leave little time for a patient, especially one who is slow to open up to an English-speaking doctor, to discuss what is really ailing him. The family member who wants her brother medicated for his aggressive behavior is going to have little patience with me methodically exploring his hallucinations, paranoia, and fears.

Often in these situations, I find that I have to remind the relative to translate, so that the conversation doesn't bypass the patient completely.

"So, Sylvan, tell me more about your memory problems," I asked the nonagenarian Russian man sitting across from me. I speak about 50 words of Russian, most of them either foods or animals, so while I had been able to win his favor by greeting him formally and directing a couple parts of a physical exam in Russian, I was dependent on translation from his son.

"He doesn't even remember if he had breakfast this morning," answered Sylvan's son immediately. "Can't remember to take his medication, can't remember anything."

I tried again. "Is this true, Sylvan?"

"What, you think I'm lying to you?" his son said, put out that I was not taking his word for it. "He needs that medicine, that Aricept, so he can remember better."

"I understand that's what *you* are seeing—I need to know what your father is feeling."

Grudgingly, the younger man translated my previous two questions, or so I think. There were a lot fewer words than I expected. But, his eyebrows rose as the old man smiled widely at me, leaned forward to put his hand on my shoulder, and began to speak to me in a conspiratorial tone. It is the only conspiracy I've ever been a part of, and I didn't even understand what I was conspiring to at first.

Healing People, Not Patients

The embarrassed son was forced to relay to me the following: "What does he know? I don't remember breakfast, because it is the same bland thing every day—you won't let me eat anything, you doctors. Most of the time, I am still hungry. And my medicine I don't forget—I skip on purpose. Too many pills. My son, he tries to make me a model patient. Not doing me any good."

So, why would I ever use a family member to translate, if this is what happens? There's a phone on the wall in every room in my office, and I have a code for the language line that I've been told to use as often as I want. On my mobile unit, where nearly every patient I see speaks Nepali, I have a hired Nepali translator there every week to translate every visit—he's been working with me so long that he usually finishes the translation by telling me what he thinks the diagnosis is, and guessing what medication I'm planning to prescribe. With that set-up, why take the shortcut of letting a relative come between me and the real story my patient wants to tell?

Well, let's see—there are the times I wait on the phone for an hour for a translator, and no one can be found. I've taken to wondering some days whether a surprise Bhutanese-Nepali holiday was declared, and no one told me, and all the interpreters have taken off to observe it. Other times, the only interpreter I can get is one of the ones who I know insults my patients—I would rather a family member, whom, as they are probably also my patient, I can reason with and redirect, than a stranger who is a jerk.

Most of the time, however, there is a simpler reason: the patients prefer it. A woman brings her son to the doctor's visit with her, because she *wants* him to interpret, to take the burden of telling the story to a stranger off her shoulders, and to fill in the little details that she may forget, but he will remember. Occasionally, an older patient comes in with a grandchild; I once got through a whole visit before realizing that the translator was only 12. She had been so tall, mature, and well-spoken that I just assumed she was an adult. One of the best translators I've ever used was a 13-year-old Korean-born girl who came in with her mother, right after I began my career and before the language line was fully operational; she was better at asking clarifying questions and patiently educating her mother than most doctors I know.

It's not only immigrants who find family members speaking for them, and often telling a much different story than they would tell themselves, when they seek medical care. Sylvan could just as easily have been an English-speaking senior from my own neighborhood, with his version of events being dismissed by an exasperated daughter, who had her own axe to grind about medications, or falls, or her father's incorrigible personality. "Dad, are you listening to what the doctor is telling you?" she might say, snapping at him, while trying to make an alliance with me. Now, the tragedy of dementia makes it essential that I get family members in the room to fill in blanks left by the patient's departing memory. Too often, though, those others who are present begin to eclipse the patient who is *supposed* to be at the center of the conversation.

Medical appointments like this can be a microcosm of an elderly person's entire life. The songwriter John Prine described it as, "Waiting for someone to say, 'Hello in there.'" In the process of slowly having to withdraw from work, from social activities, from active life, a person's world can constrict to a nondescript home that isn't really home, and a series of medical visits. If that person comes to see me and even I can't make a point of connecting with their soul, then is there really room for a soul in their body at all?

There is a strong sense among many physicians that we have medicalized old age to the point where the goal is no longer living well but staying "safe." If I'm going to set a different agenda with my older patients than just keeping them safe, I need to be able to set that agenda with *them*, not with their granddaughters or sons.

I often have the same issue at the other end of the age spectrum, by the way. It's odd, as a pediatrician (I am board certified in both pediatrics and internal medicine, so I see everyone from birth to the century-plus crowd), to think about children being strangers in the medical system. The problem is one of overlapping roles: I am supposed to advocate for the child, and so are the parents.

Unfortunately, my advocating for the child means trying to get the child to tell me the story of what's wrong from their perspective, while the parent often understands their role as needing to tell me the story *for* the child, so that they don't get it mixed up. I ask a question directly of the child, and the parent answers before the child has a chance to breathe. This is especially true when I have a translator on the phone, who can't see at which person I'm looking.

On occasion, even if I tell the translator, "I'm asking the child," or use the child's name and hear the translator address the child directly, the parent will answer. Either way, I lose the child's own perspective, even though the visit is supposed to be about them. In residency, I was taught that a child older than their fourth birthday is usually old enough to give their own history, even if the parents need to corroborate afterward. On the other hand, I see this issue cropping up as old as 13 or 14, if I don't stubbornly intervene.

Of course, the child is often to blame.

"Danny, what's wrong."

Silence.

"Joey, when did you bump your head."

Shrug.

"Angela, where does your stomach hurt?"

"It hurts, um, it … Mommy can you tell him?"

The young and old alike often default to letting someone else do the talking for them. I was always trained that adolescent exams should take place with the parent out of the room, for confidentiality reasons. As I've been in practice longer, I've realized there is actually a much more compelling reason to get the parents out of the room. Even if the teenager isn't having sex, isn't smoking, and isn't risking arrest by shoplifting, by depriving her of the "out" of turfing the question to her mother, I teach that 14-year-old girl to take responsibility for her own health. She is no longer a pre-person who is her parents' responsibility, and I no longer address my sage advice about diet, exercise, sleep and safety to them. I'm talking to her directly, about concerns that she raised to me, and getting her to take ownership of the conversation, the way she does of her friends, her phone, her room, and her "alone time."

The logical conclusion of this approach is that recently, when I've diagnosed a couple of adolescents with prediabetes, I haven't called their parents to tell them—I contact the teen directly, find out their treatment preferences, and work with them to create a follow-up plan, just like I would with an adult. I get the parents on the phone at the end to give a brief explanation and get consent for treatment. By the time I get to this stage, I'm usually comfortable with the teen themselves giving the full explanation to the parent of what needs to happen. In a world where teens are increasingly designing their own academic programs, doing more sophisticated, independent work with technology, and taking on more serious mental, physical, and skill-based challenges, I can't see continuing to treat them as little kids up until the age of consent.

With my older patients who wish to defer to their kids to speak for them, I've had to take a more nuanced approach. Fifteen years ago, after my first medical ethics course in medical school, I got into a huge shouting match with my father-in-law over the dinner table. At issue was whether doctors always needed to reveal to patients everything about their condition, even if the news was terrible—a terminal diagnosis, for example. Within the previous two years, he had lost his mother to brain cancer and his brother to stomach cancer, and he shared with me that in both cases he had not told them their diagnoses or outlook directly, but that the doctors had given him the news, and he had kept it to himself.

I lost it. This was a gross violation of the patient's autonomy, I protested. They had both had a right to know what was going on with their own bodies, so that they wouldn't become bit players in their own process of medical decisions, being shuffled around and subjected to all sorts of suffering, without full knowledge or true consent. To use the example we always bring up in the end-of-life work I do, how do you withhold from someone intelligent and literate (my wife's grandmother was, ironically, a neuropathologist in the Soviet Union, before coming to the United States in her old age) that they have cancer, when every week you are taking them to a doctor's visit at the Fox Chase *Cancer Center*?!?

I do not know what my father-in-law said to me next, but my wife does, and I'm sure it translates to something like, "Stupid, naïve American upstart, who isn't even a doctor and doesn't know what is about to hit him!" It took me the rest of medical school, all of residency, and three years in practice to realize he was right. The American medical idea of patient autonomy can itself force a kind of independence on a patient that they don't want. Really respecting the humanity of a person who is seriously ill, aging, and maybe dying actually requires questioning even a more basic assumption than what they want to do about the illness—it requires asking how much they want to know.

I remember the day my father-in-law finally won the argument. I was in the noisy hallway of 6 Main, gowning and gloving to enter a patient's room with a heavy burden in my heart. An elderly woman from Bhutan was inside, as yet unaware that her gallbladder, removed so tidily and quickly just a few days earlier, had in fact been riddled with cancerous tumors, a near-guarantee of death from cancer in the coming months. She was as yet unaware, because it would be my job to tell her.

With one gloved hand, I raised the left-hand receiver and dialed, punching the code for Nepali and waiting for the interpreter to answer. As I passed the right handset to the patient, I had a mental tickle, an uncomfortable feeling that I was forgetting something.

"*Namaste*, Indra-gi," I started. "I have some news to share with you from your—" and then I stopped. I had realized what I was forgetting. "—surgery. However, I know that many people from your country when they are older prefer for their children to discuss such things with the doctor." Her son stood in the corner, nodding; he had been hoping to head me off before coming in the room, but I had made straight for the bedside. "Is that what you would want me to do?" I asked.

She craned her neck into the phone, wrinkling her brow at the distant, tinny voice of the interpreter. Eventually, apparently satisfied that she had heard him, she nodded.

"Yes," she replied, "tell my son everything. He will understand what I want, and in any case you are the doctor, and you know what is best for me."

I began to reach for her handset to pass it to Bal, her son, when I remembered that one more question needed to be asked.

"Do you want to hear what I am telling him? Should we discuss it here in this room?"

She shook her head. "I do not need to know. Bal will take care of everything for me."

It had taken me 10 years, but I now understood what my father-in-law was saying. In the land of illness, everyone is a stranger. Some choose to approach that strangeness by achieving mastery, but for others, the strangeness is simply overwhelming, and abdicating responsibility to a trusted loved one can provide immense comfort. Whether that loved one is an oldest son, like Bal, or a brother who is trained in medicine, like my father-in-law (and his other brother, who also went into the family business), they provide a dose of familiarity and a sense that someone is looking out for everything.

Healing People, Not Patients

In between the old and the young, and among both English-speakers and immigrants, I care for many people who are estranged from me, their stories hidden from me due to mental impairments. Some are intellectually disabled, others mentally ill, and others "on the spectrum," afflicted with autism or one of its sister disorders, but the common denominator is that their communication is impaired enough that others in their circle feel the need to do their communicating for them.

Some of these folks can truly only manage to smile at me, hold my hand, high-five me or hug me. Others animatedly engage me in conversation with such prosody and emphatic gestures that I think it is me who has the communication disorder, and if I only listened more attentively and patiently I'd break through. This includes patients whose speech therapists "signed off" when they reached adulthood, saying they had reached a plateau and no longer "qualified for services," because insurance doesn't cover therapy to maintain function. Not surprisingly, I don't think the insurance sees the soul of these young adults, because eight or nine years on, I am *certain* there has been progress, actual words where there were grunts, full sentences where I used to only get a single sound before they would turn away, distracted. Someday, before I retire, I will get to know what's really going on inside their minds.

Others communicate just fine—but only amongst themselves. The deaf community has developed so much cohesion that it has its own organic culture, complete with language, slang, theater groups, and a distinct personality. And a near complete lack of reliable medical care, because delivering good care to a deaf patient who signs requires a highly trained and very expensive sign language interpreter. My partner signs—and in fact worked her way through medical school as an interpreter—and, as a result, cares for much of the deaf population of Western Pennsylvania. She is the only family physician who signs in this half of the state.

Still others are trapped inside by their disordered thought, whether the eerie hallucinations of schizophrenia or the hyper-realistic visions of post-traumatic stress disorder. They can't clear away enough of the fog, or suppress enough of the fear, to meet my eyes, arrange their words coherently, or form a clear picture of their needs, so I can help them. They, too, depend on interlocutors, friends, and family who often can't act in their best interests because *they don't know what those interests are*! They have to guess—is safety the priority? Independence? Staying off the powerful antipsychotic medications, even though they might ease the grip of the hallucinations?

My friend Jamie used to work in mental health advocacy and introduced me to the concept of a mental health advance directive. Just like an end-of-life advance directive, an MHAD allows a person to spell out values and wishes ahead of time, and designate a person to carry out those wishes. Unlike a traditional advance directive, however, the document doesn't activate with the onset of a terminal illness. When a person loses, even temporarily, the ability to make clear judgments about their own medical and psychiatric care, the agent takes over decision-making and helps to shepherd the person through a period of psychosis, catatonia, or panic. When the fog lifts, the MHAD inactivates until the next crisis, and the person becomes sovereign once again, but instead of having been a lost stranger during the crisis period, they have been under the care of their own hand-picked representative.

Even when there are no language barriers, no cognitive deficits, and no systematic dismissal of someone's wishes due to age, a person can still be a stranger, or feel like one, when they come to seek my advice.

Deonna came to see me on a Friday morning a few years ago. She painted a detailed picture of a chaotic life very quickly—inside of five minutes, I understood that she lived in one of the distressed communities across the bridge, not exactly homeless, but one missed rent or utility payment away from it. She was pretty much alone: grown kids, two husbands dead (one violence, one heart attack), and not exactly paranoid, but definitely didn't trust her neighbors, whom she referred to as "shady" or "shifty," I can't recall which. She gave careful attention to her hygiene, but not so much to her medical care, owing to not trusting doctors any more than she did her neighbors. As a result, she hadn't been in to see anyone in about 10 years, and told me I shouldn't bother getting in her business about mammograms, cholesterol, or colonoscopies, just get to the bottom of what ailed her and move on.

Deonna unsettled me, and not because she was so suspicious of my profession, but because I remember once being on the brink of homelessness myself. I was living on a very small fixed income in Israel, in my early 20s, and sharing an apartment with two friends. The week after we moved in, after my small room on the kibbutz where I had previously lived was already occupied by someone else, our short-tempered landlord called us in mid-conniption. "What are you doing, trying to cheat me! You wrote the check wrong, you forgot to put the slashes on the front, the bank won't take it, your money isn't any good. I want you and your stuff on the sidewalk by 9 a.m. tomorrow!"

Apparently, the archaic banking system in 1990s Israel required us to put a series of hieroglyphic markings on the front of the check prior to handing it to the landlord. It took almost as much effort to cash a check as to apply for a mortgage. Three of us, all Americans who foolishly thought writing a check meant filling in the name of the payee, an amount of money, and signing it, couldn't figure out how to make it work, and now, he was about to kick us out—and demand the guarantor money that older, better established friends had needed to promise on our behalf in case we blew up the apartment (which, for reasons I won't discuss, was actually a legitimate concern at that point in time). By far the most high-strung of the three, I panicked. I had no idea where I'd go, how I'd get my stuff out of there, or whether this meant my whole grand plan of living there was a failure. It felt like rock bottom.

Deonna, I knew from conversations with other folks I cared for from her community, was battling an equally arcane system, trying to balance payment plans for her water, electric, and gas bills with rent payments, keep current on her furniture lease, since she could never scrape together quite enough to buy, and keep safe in the meantime, given

Healing People, Not Patients

that petty crime went on right outside her door all the time. Homeless meant that even the flimsy front door and questionable roof that kept out thieves and thunderstorms would be gone, and she'd be living right in the thick of the danger. I didn't have an easy answer for her, but I was certainly ready to hear her story.

It wasn't a difficult story to figure out, either. She had been avoiding the dentist as assiduously as she avoided the doctor, and one of her upper right bicuspids had gone bad—very bad, as I learned during physical exam. That was probably six months ago; within two or three months after that, lightning bolts of pain started discharging dozens of times every day across her right cheek, jawbone, and lower eye socket. People told her that her face would contort into bizarre expressions every time one of these jolts let loose—the classic *tic doloreaux*, "painful tic," known in medical terms as trigeminal neuralgia. Deonna's symptoms were textbook, as was the history of a dental problem preceding the pain by some length of time.

Trigeminal neuralgia has a well-known treatment, any one of a handful of drugs usually used to control seizures, most often one called oxcarbazepine. It requires some monitoring, checking to make sure that the patient's sodium levels aren't falling too low, but otherwise is a safe and very effective treatment. I was almost excited as I described to Deonna the treatment I was proposing. For all of her insoluble problems, here at least was one that had a clear-cut answer, and since she was on Medicaid she'd even be able to afford it.

"You white doctors are all the same," she fumed. I was shocked—I didn't have any idea where this was coming from. We had talked calmly for a good 20 minutes about her situation, and I had been openly empathetic, even mentioning at some point that I had nearly been there myself (I left out the part about the check, and the explosions), and I hadn't brought up race at all, nor had she. But, she was bringing it up now.

"I came to you 'cause I'm in pain, and you're givin' me seizure drugs? You're not going to experiment on *me*! If I was white, you'd be giving me OxyContin or something right away, but 'cause I'm a black lady, I must not be in pain, and you can give me whatever you want, can't you?"

I had to check myself—was I doing something differently? TN definitely should NOT be treated with narcotics—because of the way narcotics can heighten sensitivity to pain in the long run, and because TN is already a condition where people are hyper-sensitive to painful (and hot and cold) stimuli, narcotics actually make it worse.

Oxcarbazepine is the first-line treatment, and I wasn't even trying to cut corners on cost by using an older, cheaper drug, like carbamazepine, that has worse side effects and requires more monitoring. I had seen three other cases exactly like hers recently, one of them white and the other two Nepali, and used the same drug on all three with success. I was very sure I wasn't short-changing Deonna. And I didn't think she was drug-seeking, since she hadn't asked for pain meds, only mentioning them after I had already outlined a plan. I did check afterward and found I was correct; no string of ED visits for morphine or lengthy pharmacy records of opiate prescriptions. Furthermore, even if she had been, I had certainly turned away a long line of white patients trying to score hard drugs (more on that in the next chapter). I was an equal opportunity refuser of opiates.

But, none of that mattered. Deonna had come in expecting two things, which were almost mutually exclusive: pain medication that she recognized as such, or substandard, condescending treatment, specifically because of her race. Never mind that in her condition, getting pain meds would have been substandard treatment, maybe designed to just get her to go away. She had expectations, and I was meeting the second one brilliantly by not meeting the first.

That second expectation had plenty of evidence behind it, whether it was Tuskegee, or the endless stream of literature showing that even after adjusting for economic status, African-Americans get lower quality care for a wide range of conditions than white Americans or Asian-Americans (Latinos share the disadvantage, though not always to the same degree). Most tellingly, a couple years after this event, my morning e-mail brought me a study that demonstrated that African-American children with appendicitis were less likely to get pain medication than matched white children in pediatric emergency rooms in the United States. Apparently, across the board, the medical system recognizes pain more readily in white patients than black.

The prayer that hangs above my desk (probably written by Marcus Hertz, an 18th century German-Jewish physician, but widely and erroneously attributed to Moses Maimonides) asks for the merit "to look at all who suffer, who come to seek my advice, as human beings, without difference between rich and poor, friend and enemy, good or bad, but in their suffering (pain) show me only the person." How can I, or any other physician, achieve that if there is some systematic failing that prevents us from seeing the same kind of pain equally in two people of different skin tones? And even if *I* don't do that (and believe me, I have been watching myself like a hawk since that day), the perceptions that this kind of discrimination happens are so deeply ingrained, and well-justified, that it will take lifetimes to rebuild enough trust so that Deonna and others in her situation don't walk into my exam room expecting to walk out disappointed.

Expectations are another piece of Lifeworld data that we often forget to collect. Maybe the conversation would have ended differently if I had asked Deonna something like this:

"Deonna, I think I know what the problem is, and what needs to be done to treat it, but before we talk about this, can you just tell me what you were hoping to get from this visit? What I mean is, are you looking just to know what's wrong, looking for a cure, or just looking for some temporary relief of the pain? I may not be able to do exactly what you want, but it would help me to know how to explain this to you, so I'm meeting your needs—just like it helped me to know that you weren't interested in preventive care, so I don't bother you about mammograms today."

"I just want to be out of pain, but I know ya'll not going to prescribe me any real pain meds—I know how it is with patients my color, thinking we're all drug addicts. I'm not, you know."

"It actually didn't even occur to me to think you were an addict—this is a really painful condition, and your case is classic. What do you mean when you say 'real pain meds?'" Even though I know what she means, I want to draw that out, to be absolutely clear about the expectation.

"Oh, come on, doc, don't be dumb. I mean pain meds. Morphine. You know."

"Sure, I get it. I know doctors that would probably do that, but more to avoid an argument with you than anything else. The weird thing about the condition you have is that morphine can actually make it worse—remember how sensitive you were to hot and cold, or any light touch on your face? Morphine will get rid of the ache in your tooth, but the nerve pain would actually get *worse*. You need meds for nerve pain—something a lot stronger than morphine, but in a different way. I'll also send you to the dentist next door—he's part of our health center, so I can get you in for an emergency visit today—and if *he* thinks you need a few days of Vicodin, I trust him to do the right thing. Long term, though, these other meds are better. Remember how your friends told you your face was twisting up? This disease is a lot like having seizures, just only in your face. That's why those meds work; they get the nerves in the face to calm down, just like they calm the nerves in someone's brain when they have epilepsy."

There's no way I would have undone Deonna's suspicion in a 30-minute visit, but getting her to put that expectation on the table early would have allowed me to confront it ahead of time, instead of stepping on it like a landmine. As it was, she didn't feel she could trust me anymore than the young Pakistani man trusted his interpreter. We were the enemy, part of the problem and not the solution.

At this point, I want to be clear about something. It's not every doctor that is sub-consciously racist, or dismissive of patients who are mentally ill, or condescending to the elderly or the young, or impatient with those who speak limited English. Rather, it happens often enough that all of us need the humility to be *on guard* for the possibility that we are falling prey to those prejudices and habits. Empathy is easy, when we can see the patient's humanity by looking in the mirror. It's a lot harder, when we can only see it by looking deep within ourselves.

Patients like Deonna, carrying the anger of centuries of discrimination against African-Americans, are not the only ones with a deep distrust of the medical system. I see it in some of the immigrants I care for as well, like the man who kept his epilepsy so carefully hidden. For starters, revealing a disease can sometimes ruin a person's life, if a doctor isn't careful with the information—and epilepsy is a great example. It pits doctor against patient over one of the great freedoms in modern society—a driver's license. I am the bad guy who has to ground people from driving when they have seizures—and if I don't take their licenses, I can lose mine. It is only my appeal to their own sense of fear at having an accident, or of fatally injuring another human being and carrying that guilt, that has any chance of making it common cause, rather than my livelihood over theirs.

Doctor visits like that are like the old government physicals at Ellis Island, checking new immigrants from Europe to determine if they were fit enough to enter the US. People faked their way through eye charts to hide evidence of glaucoma, distracted examiners to do all of the dexterity testing with one hand, so their withered left arm wouldn't attract attention, and suppressed tremendous pain in order to appear more vigorous than they had felt in years.

Entire lives had to be hidden sometimes. My father's best friend talks about how his father was "born in England," when in fact he was born just before boarding the ship from Russia to England, then hidden under his mother's overcoat for two days. When the ship set sail, only then did she make a tremendous show of labor pains and "deliver" a two-day old infant boy, "born" on a British sailing vessel and therefore a subject of the British Crown from birth. God Save the King!

To people who have been through exams like this, as many of my patients have in the refugee camps, my detailed, patient questioning can seem like a game of "gotcha." They have not yet developed the trust in me to know that I am on their side, 100 percent. Some large part of them still sees the medical visit as a potential trap, an obstacle to finally settling down in the promised land of America. I may be welcoming the strangers—but the strangers do not yet feel welcome.

There are sicknesses, however, that carry stigma unrelated to whether a person can drive a car, or work a particular job, or be allowed into a country. The archetypal stigmatized illness is leprosy, whether in its biblical incarnation or the way it is treated in countries around the world, even ones to which the Hebrew Bible is a late arrival. And, if we take leprosy as archetypal, we learn a few things about what happens when a person has a stigmatized illness.

First off, a person with a stigmatized illness is usually blamed in some way for getting that illness. People in the bible afflicted with leprosy were thought to have caught it as a punishment for spreading gossip. Today, we might think of lung cancer as having that stigma, the shame of having continued to smoke for years, despite "everyone knowing" that smoking is bad, often overshadowing any support or empathy the doctors have to offer. I've had patients so disgusted with the constant discussion of their past smoking that they began to disbelieve everything the oncologist said to them.

Second, a person with a stigmatized illness finds themselves shunned, cast out from society into a leper colony. Mental illness and even traumatic brain injury fall into that category today. Neighborhoods band together to keep much needed group homes "out of their backyards." Mentally ill individuals become the scapegoats for mass shootings—not that I advocate the sale of guns to the severely mentally ill, but

---

Healing People, Not Patients

rather that the only time the suffering of the severely mentally ill makes headlines is when a sufferer turns violent, rather than the much more frequent occurrences when a sufferer is themselves violently attacked. And, on a personal level, the mentally ill find themselves isolated and abandoned, because it is just plain difficult to spend time with them, dancing carefully around delusions and odd habits and rumination to try to have a "normal conversation."

Third, there is a real sense that the disease will spread like a plague, as though the victims are somehow like Camus' rats, and a tremendous mythology of how the disease spreads develops, out of any proportion to the real danger. Leprosy sufferers have traditionally inspired far more fear, for example, than people infected with the related mycobacterium that causes tuberculosis, or "consumption." In fact, a young woman with consumption was often a tragic, romantic figure in 19th century literature (think of Nicole Kidman's character in *Moulin Rouge*), even though mycobacterium tuberculosis is *incredibly* contagious and one of the most consistently deadly diseases known to man.

The modern mythology that most resembles that around leprosy is that which sprung up around HIV/AIDS when it was discovered in the early 1980s. I was a teenager, writing for my school newspaper, when 11-year-old Ryan White was being ostracized from public swimming pools in his hometown of Kokomo, Indiana, because people assumed that if he swam there he would infect the whole town. I was a college sophomore when I came into lunch one day and found a friend of mine in tears, because his childhood hero, Earvin "Magic" Johnson, had been diagnosed with HIV—and the response from his fellow players, many of them close friends on opposing teams, whom he was known to hug after they had played against each other, was to refuse to play on the same court with him, so he couldn't bleed on them. I was a senior in college when Tom Hanks played a gay man with AIDS in the movie *Philadelphia*, which depicted him being fired from his job by bosses too afraid of the disease to even sit at the same end of the conference table with him.

I was born in 1973, so the AIDS epidemic has unfolded entirely in my lifetime. By 2008, my last year of residency, the fear and mythology had been replaced by something else—perseverance. The development of potent, widely available drugs, made affordable by a fund named after Ryan White, turned HIV in America into a chronic disease, resembling diabetes or chronic kidney failure, as I described in Chapter 3..

Yet, in other parts of the world, especially Southeast Asia and sub-Saharan Africa, entire nations continue to be ripped apart by HIV. Not coincidentally, the mythology in those parts of the world is still strong, including the still prevalent view (once encouraged by the former president of South Africa, Thabo Mbeki) that HIV virus doesn't really cause AIDS, or that it is being deliberately spread by westerners, or that condom use doesn't prevent it—or that "real men" don't wear condoms. At latest report, young women are taking the rather extreme step of going on pre-exposure HIV drugs to protect themselves against the disease, since their boyfriends won't.

A lot of the stigma attached to HIV stemmed from the fact that it was first discovered in a stigmatized community—among gay men in San Francisco. For people who believed that a homosexual lifestyle was evil, here was all the proof they needed that God was punishing people for their sins by afflicting them with an illness that made them waste away from full health to emaciated, painful death in a matter of less than two years. When other cases began to pop up among drug users, or among heterosexuals in lower class minority neighborhoods, or in the "Third World," it was easy to extend the "blame the victim" logic to these other lifestyles.

Even beloved celebrities like Johnson, actor Rock Hudson, or musician Freddy Mercury didn't turn the tide. Either they were also gay, or in Johnson's case so promiscuous that "they had it coming." Ryan White's highly publicized case, because his only sin was being born with hemophilia, was the first turning point for the disease toward being treated like a mainstream illness, instead of a criminal misdeed. Likewise, tennis player Arthur Ashe, who contracted HIV from a blood transfusion during open-heart surgery, became a powerful advocate against the stigma, just as he had been an advocate for racial integration in his sport before that.

The HIV epidemic was only the latest insult visited on the LGBTQ community by medical science. HIV was identified in 1981. Up until eight years before that, homosexuality was considered a mental illness by the American Psychiatric Association. Perhaps, they were somewhat confused by the alarmingly high rate of suicides, anxiety, and depression in a community whose members needed to live dual lives, or underground existences, to avoid destroying the sham marriages that gave them respectability, escape arrest for "immorality" in cities across the Western world ("Ballad of Reading Gaol" was written after playwright and poet Oscar Wilde failed to escape such an arrest in turn-of-the-20th-century England), or duck physical violence from homophobic neighbors and classmates.

The change in classification didn't change much. LGBTQ individuals continued to be the last legitimate punching bags of raunchy humor, long after it was no longer socially acceptable to make racist, anti-Semitic, or sexist jokes, or disparage people with disabilities. As recently as 2000, Ellen DeGeneres nearly destroyed her TV career by "coming out" on her show, only to have it summarily cancelled after advertisers bailed out on her *en masse.*

Medically, this meant sub-standard treatment. Like issues of race, doctors were no less likely to be homophobic or critical of homosexuality than anyone else, though certainly not all were. Revealing your sexual orientation meant risking having that information show up on a document that would reach your employer—or your insurer, who might then decide that a gay customer was too "high-risk" and drop your policy or raise your rates. *Not* revealing it meant not discussing painful sexually transmitted infections or mental stress from fraying relationships or too many internalized secrets.

Sometimes, it was easier not to go to the doctor at all. My first week of medical school, our school's chapter of the American Medical Student Association (AMSA), led a workshop in which they encouraged students to wear rainbow pins and talked about putting rainbow stickers in offices as a signal to LGBTQ patients that these were people they could talk to safely—because the unspoken assumption at the time was that otherwise, they could not count on such understanding. It is fate, not luck, that one of the students who ran that workshop now shares an office with me.

Worst of all, the widespread perception that a gay lifestyle wasn't a legitimate family structure followed people to death's door. My friend Gary once shared with me that, "The State of Indiana determined that David and I were not fit to be parents," when they tried to adopt a child. They were not considered fit to marry at that time, either. Furthermore, that meant that should one of them fall severely ill, as Gary did several times, David might not be considered fit to serve as his next-of-kin or power of attorney. The partner he had loved for 20 years might be turned away at the door of the waiting room with the curt words, "Sorry, immediate family only," and have to wonder if they would ever get to see each other again.

I'd like to think that, like the HIV epidemic, the tide has turned for LGBTQ people as well. Surveys of younger Americans seem to show that an overwhelming majority of teens simply don't care about the sexual orientation of their friends and classmates. Media depicts positive, loving relationships among people of the same sex—or rather, depicts *normal* relationships, with the same kinds of love, abuse, conflict, reconciliation, and romantic tension that heterosexual relationships have. And politically, a lawyer who grew up in my neighborhood and went to my high school (and my synagogue) led a successful, 30-year fight to secure the right to marry for any two people who love each other enough to want to do so—including, finally, Gary and David.

The tide, however, hasn't turned for my patient Sri. When I ask my Hindu patients about sexual orientation, they chide me gently, "Oh, doctor, we don't have that in our country." It's almost worse than ostracism or harassment—it's a complete denial that such a thing as homosexuality can exist. It is exactly the way Purna described being a refugee—if you are gay, you are nowhere. Sri was a young married man, maybe in his early 20s, from northern India, I can't remember which state, and something about his story of urinary problems wasn't making any sense. I put the question to him two or three times in different, non-threatening ways, until finally, almost inaudibly, he acknowledged that he had indeed been with a male partner, at least a few times, earlier that year. Each time I see him now, his eyes beg me not to bring it up again—and never to tell his wife or parents. He will not mention the issue out loud again.

Emir wasn't so lucky either. I first saw him probably seven years ago, and he had no issue bringing up his sexual orientation; in fact, it was essential to the visit. He needed to show me his scars, both the physical and the emotional ones, and document them for his asylum hearing. Back in his native Turkey, when someone in his family "outed" him publicly, he was attacked by relatives and essentially tortured—beaten, humiliated, and subjected to such painful, deliberate injuries to his genitals that I nearly had to run out of the room a few times during the interview because I couldn't bear to listen to the story any longer. He himself seemed to be barely holding it together, except that the process of showing me the irregular pink lines on his back and bizarre patterns on his genitals were a type of vindication to him, a sign that finally someone had recognized his suffering, taken his side, and given him hope. I found out much later that an old friend of mine from high school was at that exact moment in the midst of a 10-year battle to get the US State Department to recognize persecution due to sexual identity as a legitimate reason to seek asylum in the US. We hadn't seen each other in 10 years at that point, but somehow, we managed to team up to give Emir a chance at a peaceful life.

That same friend gave me a window into the challenges faced by another group who feel like strangers in the healthcare system, namely transgender individuals. I've been using the blanket term LGBTQ, as many people do in this day and age, but especially in healthcare, the experience of a transgender person is quite different than that of a clearly identified male or female who is gay or lesbian.

Being transgender is a flashpoint in society at large right now. The simple decision of which bathroom to use is not even a conscious issue for most of us, but for transgender individuals, it is often a struggle as they decide where they belong during their time of transition. Up until recently, however, these decisions happened where any decision about where someone should pee ought to happen—in the person's own private thoughts. Very few of us have ever needed to negotiate our way to a toilet. Now, it has become a public issue so divisive that it has changed the location of the NBA All-Star Game, re-routed Bruce Springsteen's concert tour, and driven patronage of major retailers. The quiet town of Kenosha, WI, came under the microscope because of its handling of the issue. Imagine for a moment how you would feel if your right to urinate without fear of reprisal were being called into question in the national media, and you understand why a transgender person might feel like a stranger in their own hometown.

Medicine is no better. Since first year gross anatomy, my colleagues and I have learned to label things—is that an artery, or a vein? Does this count as a fever, or not? Does this person meet criteria for lupus, or do they have undifferentiated connective tissue disease?

Having to ask someone a question about whether they identify as a man, a woman, or something else, or by what pronoun or name they wish to be addressed, questions that we instinctively think should be obvious, is baffling enough. But having to recognize that there may not even be a discreet answer, but rather something along a continuum, and not necessarily even at a fixed point on that continuum, throws our organized minds into turmoil. Doctors can get so preoccupied with "genital identity" as to forget about the person's actual identity, which may not match their external appearance.

Often, we liken one stigmatized illness to another. So it is that we often refer to people who have an illness where they are shunned (think children in school with head lice) as "being treated like lepers." With sexual and gender identity issues, the pattern has been to label people who don't fit the convention as being mentally ill. Homosexuality, in general, was "un-labeled" in 1973. Being transgender, however, didn't stop being considered a disorder ("gender identity disorder") unto itself until 2013, when the most recent iteration of the Diagnostic and Statistical Manual (DSM-V) was released. Even then, the distress of being transgender and not having one's identity correlate with one's body is still considered a mental illness, called "gender dysphoria." Perhaps some of the dysphoria comes from having to negotiate one's way into the restroom.

Clearly, being harassed about toileting is preferable to mortal danger, but neither helps a person feel wholly human. I realize that the same received traditions that give us such lofty ideals as the divine origins of humanity and love for our neighbors are the same ones that demonize homosexuality. Yet, even in houses of worship that believe these things, there is often space made for LGBTQ persons to worship freely, openly, and welcomed by the other congregants. Other traditions are grappling with how to continue to regard their writ as holy, while incorporating science's new understanding of what it means to be LGBTQ. It is time for medicine to reimagine itself in the same way, and be equally welcoming of a population who have been strangers too long—especially since our inability to see their humanity for so long has caused so much harm.

The challenge of welcoming those who feel they are nowhere is why I work where I work. I come from a long line of people who have been strangers in a long line of places. We are supposed to understand how it feels to be shut out, demonized, misunderstood, or simply ignored, even if today, we live in neighborhoods where our religious symbols are displayed as prominently as the Christian ones, and you can walk down the street and tell it's Rosh Hashanah by the smell of brisket and matzah ball soup following you for seven blocks. And, we are supposed to turn that understanding into action.

The concept of a Community Health Center or Federally Qualified Health Center is that anyone who is a stranger to the healthcare system, who has to clear high barriers in order to access care, should be welcomed in and have help knocking down those barriers. As much fun as it might be, we don't use sledgehammers or explosives to take down the barriers. We use translators, the mobile medical unit, a sliding fee scale that makes care affordable for even the most destitute, rooms that accommodate a wheelchair and tables that allow for easy transfer *out* of the wheelchair for an exam, openness to all insurance and no insurance at all, house calls to the home-bound, integrated mental healthcare under the same roof as the medical providers, and an ever-growing team of nurses and social workers to help patients navigate the arcana of making specialist appointments, getting medications, and obtaining adaptive equipment.

Certainly, there are people in the world who have cleared these barriers themselves, who have turned being a stranger into an advantage and become "the first" or "the only" something or other. These people are heroes—but they are heroes because for ordinary people the things these heroes do are overwhelming, requiring more force of will than I think I would ever be able to generate. We do the work that we do, so that no one needs to be a hero just in order to heal their hurt.

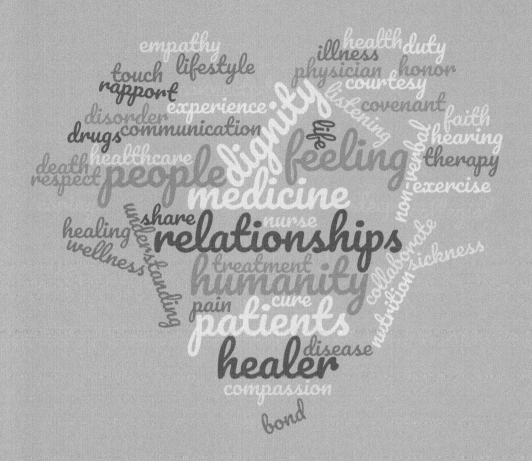

CHAPTER 8

Losing the Human Image

Sweat beaded up on the man's forehead despite the fact that it was nighttime in October. His index finger waggled as he struggled to point directly to the tip of his nose. Pinning down today's exact date was a challenge as well. He gave off an overall impression of misery.

I was new at this, having only started medical school a couple of months earlier, and it did not immediately jump out at me that I was witnessing a pretty classic case of acute alcohol withdrawal, though I knew it was likely, because I was at a Salvation Army detox clinic. My preceptor walked me through the CIWA, a scoring tool for grading the severity of alcohol withdrawal, to show me how severe this guy's symptoms really were—not bad enough to need the hospital, but definitely enough that he shouldn't go "home," wherever that was, to ride this out alone. He coached me through empathic responses to everything the man might say about why he had kept drinking, and ways to support him through his decision to quit, suddenly, so that the frightening experience of withdrawal, and possibly delirium tremens within the next day or two, didn't scare him drunk again.

He did not prepare me for rolling up the man's sleeve to take his blood pressure and finding a huge tattoo of a Nazi swastika. I have never, before or since, felt my empathy evaporate so quickly as this. I am not a vindictive person, but all I could think was, "Well, it serves him right. This is poetic justice." With no experience to draw on, I couldn't even bring myself to discuss this with the preceptor. Instead of the heartfelt discussion I was meaning to have, I finished my exam, hastily excused myself, and went to present to the attending without mentioning the tattoo, or how ill it made me feel, or the malicious thoughts it was triggering in my mind.

There are encounters in medicine that push the limits of empathy. I once asked the question, "Are there any patients in whom you have trouble seeing the divine image?" to a group of colleagues and students who were gathered for a Spirituality in Medicine retreat—a self-selected group of highly empathic healers, if ever there was one. Just as I had failed in my first attempt to muster empathy for the man wearing the swastika tattoo, I assumed that even these thoughtful, reflective people, who train others how to find compassion and empathy for their patients, might have the same struggles in their own lives. I assumed correctly.

At the top of the list were unrepentant alcoholics and patients who had abused not drugs, but other people, either their intimate partners or their children. Other colleagues expressed to me their challenges in caring for convicted pedophiles or other serious offenders, whether in the prison system or outside it. As I care for several ex-convicts myself, I know that the care afforded these patients is often, as a result, impersonal, vindictive, and substandard. Medications are continued in almost rubber stamp fashion, long past the point of utility, abnormal lab tests are ignored, and symptoms are minimized. I take these complaints with a grain of salt, since the patient is naturally bitter about having served his time, but even after discharge, well-meaning doctors outside the penal system struggle to separate the relationship that develops over repeated visits, and the trust the patient places in us, with the knowledge of what they have done to get themselves in to prison in the first place.

Several female colleagues, and a few males as well, have told me of their inability to keep the divine image in mind, when they have to worry about whether it is safe to close the door to the exam room. One receptionist I used to work with has a sixth sense for dangerous patients and used to call back to my desk to warn me, if I was going into a room where she thought I should protect myself first. I know colleagues who have been groped, intimidated, physically threatened, or actually assaulted; they find themselves suddenly identifying very closely with the victims of the patient's previous crimes, rather than empathizing with the patient. Realizing that in spite of their fear and unease, they still bear a responsibility for this person's care is a shock to their system.

Empathy is sometimes replaced by anger at patients and their family members for individual acts that seem to us to be bafflingly stupid. I spent several months of my residency in a pediatric emergency department with a number of excellent, kind, and usually unflappable attendings. On the other hand, presented with a case of a teenager injured riding an ATV, especially without a helmet, a child with spinal trauma from a trampoline, a girl who nearly drowned in an un-fenced swimming pool, or a boy bleeding from a bullet wound caused by an unsecured, poorly stored loaded firearm, they lost all self-control and all compassion for the distraught parent who failed to prevent these horrible tragedies.

In my experience, the patient behaviors that distract healers from the patients' humanity fall into three categories. The first category includes patients who have committed a crime or some other heinous act. Their behavior offends the provider so badly that they struggle to care whether the patient suffers any further, or else they believe that the suffering is deserved, like I did with the tattooed man. In the second group are those who engage in self-destructive behavior. Providers like my colleagues in the emergency medicine world find themselves endlessly frustrated trying to undo damage that they believe the patient brought on himself. The final category is those whose behaviors put them somehow directly at odds with the provider, or indeed with the whole medical establishment, by being argumentative, deceitful, accusatory, disruptive, or downright threatening to some or all of those they come in contact with. Providers for patients in this group find themselves struggling not to see the patient as an enemy or adversary, rather than as a partner as we have been describing.

We see a misshapen clavicle, a souvenir of a close encounter with the pavement that began as a 12-pack of cheap beer. Edematous legs, doughy enough to leave the imprint of a man's entire hand for a minute or more, that originated in a Doritos binge during the Steeler game. An epic cough that came to life from 80 pack-years of cigarettes and keeps getting worse with every day, in which there is "too much stress" to quit yet.

Cases like these are the people seeking care in emergency rooms, and the people who make up the bulk of primary care visits in the US, and the bread and butter of cardiologists and pulmonologists. By and large, they are the entire world. The World Health Organization's list of leading causes of death in 2012 includes only one category of diseases, diarrheal illnesses, in which individual human behavior does not play some kind of causal role. The top five (ischemic heart disease, stroke, COPD, lower respiratory tract infection, and trachea/bronchus/lung cancers) all have some relation to tobacco use, and the top two are strongly correlated with poor diet and obesity. HIV claims the most victims in parts of the world where it passes by unprotected sexual intercourse involving infected individuals unwilling to wear condoms, and road deaths clearly relate to driving behaviors, ranging from aggression to alcohol intoxication to distracted driving.

Compared to caring for children suffering from congenital illnesses, adults dying of sporadically occurring, unpredictable cancers, or epidemics of Ebola, MERS, or other scourges, the physician dealing with a patient whose woes are seen as self-inflicted is often short on empathy, or even pity. Doctors go on tirades about smoking, stupid parents, or overeating.

Yet, I know a *lot* of physicians—every single one of us has some bad habit we cannot break. My own love-hate relationship with coffee (love the taste, love the wakefulness, hate the sore throat and stomach pain) and my inability to unplug at night so I can get decent sleep are just two examples. Some of us never exercise, while others eat the same diet we subsisted on in residency (free pizza!) and expect to avoid the consequences it wreaks on our patients. Still others drink heavily, and many, especially those with easy access, like anesthesiologists, become addicted to drugs. Precious few still smoke, though once it was common to see a chain-smoking resident, with a lit butt hanging from their lips while delivering the grim news of lung cancer to a patient. Ironically, many of these habits develop as a mechanism for coping with the frustration we feel with our *patients'* bad habits and our own inability to right the ship.

For some in the medical establishment, none of this matters. They see their job as fixing the current problem, not changing the person—in other words, they are there to treat the disease, not understand the illness, or even lessen the overall sickness in society. The patient has a problem that requires a certain knowledge and expertise to solve, and they solve it. The economics of our system reward this approach greatly: a cardiologist who spends an hour in the cath lab placing four stents in a patient's heart will be able to successfully bill insurance for somewhere around $30,000, whereas that same patient's family doctor will be lucky to bill for $150 for the four 15-minute visits he spends over the following six months trying to get that patient to quit smoking.

For a lot of us, however, the frustration over avoidable, preventable diseases cannot be suppressed. It is not necessary to be perfect to rebuke someone for such behavior. If it were, no one would ever give or receive criticism, because no one would be qualified to give it. However, recognition of the flaws in our own behavior should only make us more empathetic, more understanding, when we approach someone else about their shortcomings. *How* we deliver the rebuke is as important as the fact that we deliver it at all. We can start by letting the patients who are driving us mad share their stories.

The narrative that I have heard from smokers has been eye-opening. Cigarettes are the calm at the end of the day. They are the only constant in a chaotic life. They actually produce a feeling of relaxation and clear-headedness when the smoker begins to feel overwhelmed. They are an inextricable part of coffee—of alcohol—of a good meal—of a late-night chat with a good friend—of satisfying sex.

One angry smoker I knew in college once reacted to the flippant remark that every cigarette he smoked would shorten his life by seven minutes by retorting, "If I had those seven minutes back, I'd probably use them to smoke a cigarette." An ICU nurse I worked with in residency routinely ended her overnight shifts by smoking several cigarettes (and eating three or four strips of bacon) in determination to choose an early, fatal heart attack over the slow decline into multi-organ failure of most of her patients. And one gentleman I know, unable to find the words to deliver his narrative, simply drew the pack of cigarettes out of their permanent home in his shirt pocket and gave it a loud, wet kiss. Yet, every one of them knows the truth that was obvious even before the 1964 Surgeon General's report—smoking kills.

Behavioral change can be hard. Surgeon General Luther Terry, himself, was a smoker who was asked about the habit at his news conference when the report was issued. When asked how long ago he had quit, Terry replied, "About 30 minutes ago." Still, Terry's report referred to smoking as a habit. It was not until the report of one of his successors, C. Everett Koop, in 1989, that the terminology was changed to recognize that it was, in fact, an addiction to nicotine.

The addiction language was a powerful change. About six years ago, I attended a lecture at a national medical conference about smoking cessation. The speaker described the smoker as effectively being of two minds—the rational mind, with whom the healer has the discussion about smoking cessation, the one that engages in motivational interviewing and makes constructive plans for the future, and the addict brain that second-guesses those plans, decides it is more afraid of the momentary side effects of a nicotine patch or a smoking cessation drug, and runs back into the arms of the faithful old lover, tobacco.

Yet, addicts do sometimes quit using tobacco. A relative gets lung cancer, a life milestone passes, a physical task that used to be easy suddenly makes them short of breath, and they can throw away the last pack without a second thought. Other times, they make a slow, painful separation, going from two packs, to one, to a half, with stops and starts and relapses. They quit for six months, nine months, then falter and smoke again, sometimes for a few years, before mustering the courage to try again. And, in between, they may end up in the emergency department with pneumonia, or an asthma attack, or worse, a cancer.

Healing People, Not Patients

It takes an incredible amount of forbearance to move with someone through these stages of behavior change. Nothing bothers me more than a patient who finally moves from the contemplative to the action phase of behavior change, only to fail to go to the pharmacy to pick up the prescription for nicotine patches I worked so hard to get them to accept. They do not call to tell me this. They just return six months later, with a sheepish smile on their face, a tell-tale rectangular bulge in their jacket pocket, and an unmistakable aroma from the cigarette they smoked *on my doorstep*, before checking in for their visit.

I use addiction language, rather than "habit" language, because it helps me avoid the "willpower" response. Physicians who have resisted the temptation to smoke or drink heavily, or even those who have themselves overcome addiction, can come to see those individuals who don't kick the "habit" as being weak-willed, not trying hard enough, or simply not wanting to quit. I return again and again to that lecture in Philadelphia, the one that helped me recognize that an addict doesn't always behave rationally, and that cigarettes exert a type of control in a smoker's mind that doesn't make sense to someone who doesn't smoke. There are other factors at play, however, with these behaviors that goes beyond merely the chemical hold they have on our dopamine receptors.

People who are obese, diabetic, hypertensive, or in heart failure also return again and again to the precise foods—salty, sweet, starchy, high calorie, liquid calorie, laden with trans fats—that have created and sustained their diseases, even after being "educated" in the dangers of their habitual diets. Alcoholics continue to hang out with drinking buddies and do with them what drinking buddies do. Narcotic addicts continue to visit emergency departments for "11/10 pain" and buy other people's leftover medications off the street. For many of these people, addiction is only a part of the narrative. In many cases, a system that has no particular interest in their individual well-being sets them up to fail, or, at least, erects tall barriers to their success, in service of its financial goals.

After tobacco use, the individual behavior that most affects mortality is diet, which, as previously noted, plays a major role in the genesis of the two leading causes of death on the WHO list. While the individual roles of sugar, fat, and salt in the march toward heart disease and stroke are still being worked out, most processed foods are designed to get exactly the right balance between those three items, as well as additional features like "mouth feel," to reach a "bliss point," at which people feel they can, and want to, just keep on eating the food indefinitely. The Cheeto, the Lunchable, and Cherry Vanilla Doctor Pepper are just a few examples of foods designed using this science.

None of these particularly do it for my palate, but there is a particularly ironic one that does—the ice cream at the Berkey Creamery in University Park, PA, run by students in the Penn State department of nutrition. That same department is also home to Barbara Rolls, pioneer of the volumetrics approach to weight loss, which encourages replacement of calorie dense foods—like, for example, ice cream—with bulky, low calorie foods that have similar textures—like frozen pureed bananas, or whipped egg whites. Don't try this at the Creamery, though; one ice cream cone is larger than the head of an average-sized toddler, and the only bananas are the ones being served as a topping for the ice cream itself.

However, the Creamery is a special experience—a treat worth waiting for when parents pick up their student at college, a celebration after the statistics final, or a nice ending to a first campus date. Since I live three hours away from State College, I eat there about once every two to three years.

Many other carefully processed food disasters make their way into everyday diets. Vending machines containing potato chips and packaged cookies are strategically planted in break rooms, hallways, and outside cafeterias (just in case you didn't eat enough lunch)—and labeled with stickers touting "smart choices." Prepackaged meals containing extraordinary amounts of all three of the bliss-making ingredients are hawked as being sensible solutions to the morning rush to feed hungry kids—or directly to kids as being a way to take control of lunchtime away from their parents. Potato chips, pretzels, and other junk foods are aggressively marketed to restaurants as add-ons for meals, not just snacks. The temptation is no longer a three hour drive down US 22, it is right in your face, all the time.

In particular, the products are often marketed, and priced, to appeal to people in disadvantaged communities and developing nations, which led then-Coca-Cola executive Jeffrey Dunn to remark, while on a trip to the *favelas* of Brazil, "These people need a lot of things, but they don't need a Coke." For his epiphany, and the strategic changes he suggested in its wake on his return to Atlanta, Dunn was fired from Coke.

Dunn's experience in Brazil could have been replicated in many parts of the US as well. As unhealthy foods are marketed to low-income consumers, healthy food often becomes harder and harder to find. Such a situation is called a "food desert," an area where the nearest full service grocery store or supermarket selling fresh produce is over a mile away, or more than 10 miles in a rural area.

In my home, Pittsburgh, 47 percent of the city's residents lived in a "food desert" in 2012 (about 145,000 people), of whom 71 percent were low income and therefore lacked the means, and often the transportation, to take their business elsewhere. Their only options? The corner stores, convenience stores at gas stations, and fast food restaurants, which primarily stock "bliss point" processed foods, serve French fries as their primary vegetable, and offer a wide variety of sugar-sweetened beverages in increasingly larger sizes. At least the Cokes they were planning to sell in Brazil were only 6.7 ounces, as opposed to the 20-ounce "individual" bottles now common on US shelves.

This "built environment" of food deserts and engineered bliss-inducing foods makes the willpower argument look weak. Certainly, there are those who can withstand the power of Cheetos, and those who will make the trek across the food desert to find the oasis. But, with limited means, and facing products and product placement designed to live up to slogans like, "No One Can Eat Just One," few will reach this point without a lot of help. The healer who takes the time to dig deep with the patient and uncover the specific booby traps that keep that person from eating better ("Double Stuf Oreos? Me, too! Wow, looks like we both need a good strategy. What do you think we should do about this?") or break down the obstacles to getting the food they know they need ("Two buses and 45 minutes each way to the nearest Shop n' Save? No, that *is* nuts. I wonder what options we can help you find closer to home.") will get a lot further than the one who scolds.

I may sound like I'm making excuses for my patients, and putting the onus for all behavior change on the healer and the healthcare system, and the blame for all the missteps on an environmental conspiracy. One could easily argue that most people don't need their doctor to provide them with excuses for their behavior or explanations for why they are still smoking and eating potato chips—they can do that well enough for themselves. In fact, if you ask my patients, they will tell you that I am *not* a pushover on these issues—more of a constant annoyance, but a constant annoyance with a smile and a gentle demeanor.

What my patients need is for me to validate those excuses as reasons why they have not changed their behavior, while refusing to accept those excuses as reasons the behavior *cannot* change. If I'm doing a good job using my motivational interviewing techniques, the patient might list his excuses and immediately reflect, "I guess when you say that out loud, it sounds pretty lame. I suppose I could just buy chewing gum, instead of cigarettes, the next time I go to the store and use that to keep my mouth busy when I'm nervous."

Other times, the patient will have no ready ideas for how to defuse a particular excuse, and I will suggest a strategy—only to be met by an additional series of excuses for why the *strategy* won't work. When someone moves forward with a behavior change, my job is to be their cheerleader, providing positive reinforcement (including "hard data," like lower cholesterol or better numbers on peak-flow breathing testing). When they do not move forward, it's my task to call them out on it—but to do that without shaming, without intent to harm with words, only to unpack the problem and see where the progress toward change was derailed.

So, do I ever just get to say, "I've made a good faith effort to help you, pushed myself to understand your situation, and you have not met me halfway. I can't continue knocking myself out knowing you are not fulfilling your part of the covenant. I can't help you if you won't help yourself?"

This is what I meant in Chapter 6 when I pointed out that the covenant can't be maintained by the doctor alone, and that the patient has as much responsibility in building the medical community as I do. I cannot promote health or effect healing by myself. The patients have to allow themselves to be healed—really, to do some of the healing themselves.

Many of my patients have heard me loud and clear about the need to quit smoking, and not done so—and in exchange for their inaction have accepted that I am now free to say something I don't normally say to patients, namely, "I told you so," when they develop bronchitis or worse. The covenantal relationship, built over several years, allows us to be this frank with one another. That same relationship also allows me to see that the recalcitrant smoker is not only a smoker—that this is only one of that person's problems. When we turn our attention to different issues, those discussions do not need to be colored by my frustration over their failure to quit.

Nicotine addiction is frustrating enough. The other addictions I deal with, however, create a dynamic all their own between me and my patients.

There's a call that I get a lot after hours and on weekends.

"Doctor Weinkle?"

"Yes?"

"I know it's the weekend, and I'm not supposed to be calling about this now, but here's the thing—my medication was stolen, and I need to get refills or I'm going to go into withdrawal. I don't know what I'm going to do without it."

The voice on the line is panicked, maybe even in tears. There has usually been a police report filed already, something that is mentioned explicitly three or four times in the course of the telling.

"Which medication was it?" I ask, even though I already know the answer.

"It was the Klonopin—luckily they didn't take my Seroquel or my Prozac." Sometimes, it isn't Klonopin, but Adderall, tramadol, or some other controlled substance. But, it's always something on the DEA schedules.

"I can't refill that for you over the weekend, or early. We discussed this when I first gave you the prescription—controlled substances can't be refilled early, after hours, or if they've been lost or stolen. That's a policy we've had for years, and we don't make exceptions to it."

"What am I supposed to do? How am I supposed to survive until my renewal date comes up?! I'll just have to go to the ER—do you want me to do that?"

Don't make me answer that question, please, I think to myself. Anything I say will be the wrong thing.

I have played this scene dozens of times, with dozens of patients. Every time I do, I grit my teeth, dig in my heels, and recite in a calm voice the same words: "I can't …" I never yell, I never curse, and I never insult the person or directly impugn their honesty. Yet, all the while, my head is ready to explode.

Here's the problem: I am nearly certain that each individual (and there have been many, with only minor variations on the theme) who calls me with this script is lying. I am equally certain that one day, I will refuse medication to someone who *isn't* lying.

As I mentioned when discussing smoking, an addicted brain will do backflips and tie itself in knots in order to believe that continuing the addiction makes perfect sense. That same brain, addicted to a controlled or illegal substance, rather than perfectly legal cigarettes, will invent all sorts of ideas to enable it to get a hold of that substance—or, unable to invent anything good, will reuse someone else's tired, old ideas and believe, with perfect faith, that it has stumbled upon the only remaining naïve doctor in the world who's never heard that excuse before.

Sometimes, the ruse is obvious. There's a voice in the background feeding information to the caller, who stumbles over the words and actually stops and (ineffectively) cups the phone to say, "What did you say?" or the same voice will call twice and claim to be a different person each time. Other times, though, it's easy to get swept up in the story, to begin to feel real empathy for the horrible situation this person is now stuck in.

Sometimes, the story is so poignant that I begin to remember a piece of "pain theater" one of my professors did in med school, where he had a classmate of mine portray the phenomenon of "pseudo-addiction." The pseudo-addict is really in pain, but exhibits "drug-seeking" behaviors, like repeated requests for specific meds, agitation, asking for medication earlier than scheduled, and trying multiple providers, because no one has adequately treated his pain.

When I pass a panhandler on the street I give money. On occasion, if the opportunity presents itself, I duck into a fast-food joint and buy a meal, or share my restaurant leftovers (though I know of restaurants that actively discourage this behavior to keep the homeless from congregating nearby). When I was still learning to cook and didn't know how to estimate portion sizes well, I used to bring huge pans of leftovers to where I knew the homeless of Oakland (Pittsburgh's university district) congregated. I know countless people who think I'm a sucker for doing these things, citing the likelihood that the panhandler isn't really poor, or will use the money to buy drugs, alcohol, or cigarettes, instead of food, or will just spread the word to other homeless people and make the problem worse.

When someone challenges me in that situation, I usually retort with a story from one of the Hasidic masters, whose disciples asked why he gave money to beggars, when so many of them were charlatans. He replied, "I would rather give money to 99 charlatans, so that one honest beggar should not go wanting, rather than refuse 99 honest beggars to avoid giving to one charlatan." Since I don't know who's aboveboard, there is less harm done by giving whenever I can—though I did turn away the guy in the Jerusalem bus station who tried to hit me up for money for a second time, pretending he didn't recognize me, less than five minutes after I had handed him enough to buy a full meal.

At the end of that recurring phone call, I often hang up and wonder, "Should I be following that same principle with my patients on controlled meds?" After all, many of them do need the medications they're on, completely legitimately, and, in many cases, it was at my urging that they went on them. Even more of them have lives that are in chaos, for which "real" solutions require moving heaven and earth, and therefore, by comparison, a small pill that "takes the edge off" seems like the only way to cope. Where do I get the right to suddenly turn gatekeeper and refuse those patients their medications? How am I supposed to sort out the honest from the charlatans?

Herein lies the reason that "drug-seeking" patients make physicians so angry. Three reasons, actually.

First of all, doctors, myself included, are generally smart people with big egos—or at least, people with big egos who are egotistical enough to believe that we are very smart. We do *not* like being made to look stupid or being taken advantage of. A patient trying to hoodwink us out of an extra script for oxycodone is essentially screaming at us, "I am smarter than you!"

On top of this, we are also extremely *busy* people, and we are loath to "waste" the time we must spend on the process of verifying that someone needs or deserves medication. My practice no longer prescribes "hard narcotic" pain medications—schedule II drugs such as oxycodone, morphine, or Vicodin. Part of the reason we stopped doing so was because our nursing staff was spending so much time on the due diligence of calling pharmacies, collecting urine drug screens, arguing with patients demanding increased doses or early refills, and safeguarding printed prescriptions so that they didn't leave with the patient before the prescriber's conditions were met, that they couldn't attend to the tasks of the rest of our patients. It got to the point that we were needing to find ways to outsmart the patients who had found ways to outsmart our system, like taking the temperature of urine samples to ensure that they were freshly voided from a live human body (we once got a sample that was 84 F!).

That's an admittedly selfish reason to lose sight of someone's humanity. After all, we love magicians, who make their living at fooling us. The more compelling reasons we dislike the deceitfulness of addicts are a function of the effect it has on others.

As I just mentioned, my office no longer prescribes heavy-duty narcotics. By the anecdotal evidence I get from my patients, we are far from alone in having made this decision. However, because of our frustrations with those who abused the system, the minority of patients who are in serious need of these medications now have to endure additional administrative hurdles and long waits to see overbooked and often unsympathetic pain management clinics, rather than dealing with a primary care problem, being out of pain, in a primary care setting. Even patients who do get such meds from us, such as those who have just suffered an acute fracture, have just had major surgery, or have solid organ cancer, get read the riot act prior to receiving their prescriptions.

The policy I mentioned in the aforementioned phone call scenario? It, too, was written to shut down the deceivers, by preventing them from calling after hours, when they might get a provider who didn't know them well enough to suspect, or when it would be harder for the on-call provider to check the medical record (remote access from home has proven very frustrating to such folks). And yet, this policy ends up constraining many of our behavioral health patients who can't get a hold of the refill line before 4 p.m. Friday to get their Klonopin, or our patients with ADHD who, because they have ADHD, sometimes forget to call until Saturday morning, or 9:00 on Wednesday night.

It doesn't matter that I make a point to tell everyone, even folks I *do* think are pulling a fast one, that I am not accusing *them* of pulling a fast one—they all *feel* accused. How can they *not* feel accused of dishonesty, when they know that if they come into the office to do a drug screen, *I will make my medical assistant measure the temperature of their pee, rather than take their word that the urine they are providing is their own, freshly voided sample?* After all, what kind of person carries spare or borrowed urine around with them, if they're *not* a drug addict?

At this point, it's fair to wonder why I *don't* apply the panhandler rule to prescription drugs. If I know for certain I'm causing harm even to a few people, then what's the harm in letting a few folks slip by who are up to no good?

For starters, the policy on pain meds in our office coincided with a series of publications in the medical literature that showed that chronic use of high potency opioid medications does not actually reduce pain in non-cancer pain patients. I recently spoke to a friend who is a retired anesthesiologist and pain doctor, and learned that he spent the early part of his career weaning people off of narcotics, because that was the standard of care for non-cancer pain in the 1970s and 1980s. For his few patients who had cancer-related pain, he went straight to the "big guns," usually methadone, and gave as much as people needed to relieve their symptoms. Only in the 1990s, with the rise in direct-to-consumer advertising encouraging patients to demand narcotic pain relief for their chronic pain disorders, and promising that medications like OxyContin were completely safe, did he begin getting patients in clinic asking to be put *on* heavy narcotics.

Once on these medications, people build a tolerance to these meds, develop side effects, like constipation, itching, and nausea, which then need to be treated with other medications. Taking these medications can even lead to the development of a syndrome called opioid hyperalgesia, where the narcotics make them more sensitive to certain kinds of stimuli, feeling pain from even gentle, firm touches in certain tender areas—much like Deonna in the story detailed in Chapter 7.

People do develop addiction, despite the old saw that treating pain doesn't produce addiction. Better to say that *properly* treating pain doesn't lead to addiction—which means not giving a 60-day supply of oxycodone for an injury that might require a week's worth, and not using narcotics to manage chronic, smoldering pain, but liberally giving IV pain meds to surgical patients in the hospital and liquid morphine to dying hospice patients at home. Those patients, as well as the handful who *do* need chronic narcotics, almost always need the care of an expert, just like the small percentage of patients whose diabetes I can't manage with good, standard care require an endocrinologist.

Stimulants for ADHD and sedatives for anxiety, the two other meds most often abused, are no different. There are addiction and overdose syndromes there as well, often with destructive effects on people's lives. Sedative overuse can combine in deadly mixtures with alcohol, or motor vehicles. Stimulant addiction or overuse is a cause of violent, psychotic rages that often lead to physical violence or suicide. All three categories of drugs have a street market that leads them into the wrong hands, and can contribute to addiction or death for people far removed from the original prescriber. Yet, law enforcement can and sometimes does hold the prescriber liable for drugs that they prescribed that end up trafficked illegally. At that point, the addict has not only damaged the other patients in the practice by inconveniencing them, they have also ruined the physician's good name.

Which brings me to the final point regarding deceit. At a certain point, having to play drug cop, instead of being a doctor, wears us down. The same factor is true for the nurses that I work with and the pharmacists to whom I have spoken. The result is a type of burnout that comes from loss of empathy. An empathetic physician is willing to take a patient at their word, and advocate for that patient in their hour of need. Advocacy, however, puts a physician's good name on the line with whoever we're advocating with—the pharmacy, the insurance, the DMV. The first time they get wind of a clinician's reputation being tainted by having gone to bat for a known drug-seeker or trafficker will be the last time that physician's name carries any weight. With that fear in mind, a lot of us struggle not to see each new patient who complains of severe panic attacks, claims to have undiagnosed ADHD, or waxes eloquent about their 11/10 pain everywhere as a potential trap. The work of dishonest people who have gone before has poisoned the well of our compassion for everyone who comes after.

This point doesn't only apply to situations where controlled medications are at issue. My medical license makes me the gatekeeper for all sorts of things: permission to work, permission to skip work (or school or jury duty), permission to drive and the threat of having a license taken away, certification that someone will not work for a long time, and might not even be able to take care of himself without help, fitness for *another* doctor to do surgery, and desirability to people in my father's business (life and disability insurance, thank you). The most interesting "gate" I've ever been asked to unlock with my medical key was to sign off on a handicapped parking placard for a patient with overactive bladder, so they could get to the bathroom as soon as they got out of the car.

Here, too, there are people who will try to use the system to their advantage, making it that much harder for those in genuine need. Hard as it may be for me to

---

fathom that someone would want to be declared disabled, when they are not, my colleagues and I encounter people all the time who hand us forms to complete for entitlement programs, county assistance, accessible housing, and paid caregiving to whom our first reaction is, "They want what?!?"

This situation is especially vexing, when it involves a new patient being seen initially by a new medical student, who finishes the entire presentation and then says, "Oh, and she has this form she needs you to fill out for disability," even though she has never met me before.

There are myriad reasons why people apply for disability. Cancer, end-stage or advancing organ failure, and neurological disability are some obvious ones, and fairly easy illnesses to judge a person's level of impairment. Far more common, however, are three main categories: injury, chronic pain, and mental illness. In these categories are a host of different diagnoses: back pain, neck pain, various joint injuries (from arthritis of the hips to plantar fasciitis), recurrent migraine, chronic abdominal pain, endometriosis, depression, anxiety, PTSD and bipolar disorder.

These categories contain their "no-brainers" as well. The young man I saw in the emergency department as a resident years ago who had been paralyzed by a gunshot wound to the spinal cord was clearly disabled. My patients who are nearly catatonic due to mental illness, whether from schizophrenia or trauma, are obviously disabled— though getting them the services they need for day-to-day care is especially challenging, since their illness is neither "medical" nor "intellectual disability" (formerly known as "mental retardation"). Furthermore, the handful of patients I care for whose chronic pain is at the point where they pound their own fists against the affected areas several hours a day to get it to stop are plainly disabled. Their basic activities of daily living, their relationships, and their independence in the world are so profoundly affected that there's no real doubt.

Unfortunately, most cases are not so cut and dried. What is 10/10 pain? I think of 10/10 pain as the first patient I ever saw on a surgery service in medical school, an army recruiter with a freshly ruptured appendix and a rock-hard abdomen. How do I reconcile that memory with a person calmly sitting across from me with a bored expression on his face telling me his pain is *also* 10/10? Is this person who has a college degree and has moved mountains advocating for their own care really totally disabled or just unable to do *physical* labor, but capable of working a desk job? Does this individual's bipolar disorder really constitute true disability, or has this person just gotten fired repeatedly for having incredibly poor judgment about what comes out of their mouth when speaking to supervisors? Add in the people that my colleagues and I know are drawing disability checks each month, yet also making money by doing very physical odd jobs, like painting their neighbors' garage, or even by running an online business, and it is easy to become skeptical.

Once that skepticism sets in, it colors every interaction that involves those papers, and every interaction labeled with one of those diagnoses. I have read countless articles

Healing People, Not Patients

and blog posts over the years (and sat in on more than one conversation) about "least favorite diagnoses"—and almost all of them list the aforementioned diagnoses I recounted, the common disability diagnoses that involve pain that is difficult to pin down and impairments that are hard to measure. There are still debates raging in the medical community over whether disorders like fibromyalgia, irritable bowel syndrome, chronic fatigue syndrome, and complex regional pain syndrome even exist.

I'm hard pressed to come up with a clearer way to tell someone that you think they're a faker than to tell them you "don't believe in" their diagnosis. Yet, this is the mindset many of us are in when we see people who are struggling to get by with daily pain, physical limitations, and a history of emotional challenges, workplace injury, or incomplete medical diagnoses for their ailments.

I spend a lot of my time with these people. At any given time, I could tick off a dozen names of people in emotional and financial limbo because they are too sick to work anymore, be it driving a bus, lining swimming pools in concrete, sitting still at a desk patiently calming down irate customers, or trapping rodents, yet not yet recognized as being disabled by the state or federal government. They wait and worry, without income, without a piece of their identity, because they are idle, and prior to 2015, likely without health insurance and therefore without a way to acquire further evidence of their disability by getting imaging, consultations, or physical therapy.

Why are they waiting? In part, they are victims of an inefficient bureaucracy. The government agencies handling their cases are overwhelmed with caseloads that are too big for the insufficient staff that they must process those cases. They become a case number instead of a person, though I am happy to say that in my advocacy for my patients, I have encountered a lot of really committed civil servants, who genuinely listen to their clients' stories and do their best to treat them as humans first.

A major contributor to the wait is the layers upon layers of safeguards put in place to ensure that no one "undeserving" is accidentally helped by the system. Of late, nearly every case is denied on the initial application, requiring lengthy and expensive appeals with legal representation to prove disability. Once proven, the disabled individual may have to reappear for a "functional evaluation" every few years to show that they are still disabled. My colleague's deaf patients were nearly all born deaf. Yet, periodically she is asked by the state to certify that they are still disabled, as though they may somehow magically become hearing in the meantime and are merely pretending to still be deaf.

The entire process makes me, and these patients waiting through the arduous process, angry at the folks defrauding the system. The issue arises, who are these "fakers," and why are they doing this to the poor folks I'm trying to help?

I will tell you first who they are not. They are not people lucky enough to have jobs where they can telecommute when they are sick. They are not people with five weeks of paid sick leave a year. They are not people who have workplace-based disability insurance or good workman's comp—and when they are there are plenty of barriers to them getting compensation from those sources as well, again to prevent fraud. They are not people who can easily "reinvent themselves" and change careers when they can't continue at their previous professions.

There are holes in the system that create a dichotomous situation: either you do what you already know how to do, full-time or even overtime, or you are disabled. Job retraining, like what Pennsylvania offers through its Office of Vocational Rehabilitation, is difficult to come by, and the Americans with Disabilities Act still doesn't require an employer to change things about a job that can't be changed—a housekeeper still needs to be strong enough to lift the mop bucket. Wage earners can often work for weeks at a time without a day off to be able to schedule a doctor visit, and "calling off" invites dirty looks, retributive punishment at work, being passed over for promotion, and firing.

Making "too much money" (a small fraction of federal poverty level, prior to Medicaid expansion) would mean losing medical assistance to care for the illness, which, untreated, makes it impossible to work, creating a catch 22. Most frustrating for physicians to keep straight in our cut-and-dried minds, the law defining disability under the Social Security Act allows disabled persons to work a certain limited number of hours, so long as they don't go over the limit considered "gainful employment." This last factor is, in my experience, the place where the most fraud is committed—because the alternative is either meeting the demands of an employer, who will ask much more than the person can deliver, or trying to live on $701 a month.

How do I know all this? From communicating with the people living this narrative. I don't mean to say that there are no actual cases of fraud that exist. I have encountered my share and certainly refused to submit my share of disability forms for people who were clearly gaming me and the system.

In the remaining cases, however, when a med student hands me the surprise disability form, I do what I have been advocating throughout this book: get the story. Not only the story of "Why do you feel you can't work?" but also the story of the impact of the complete process on the person's life. Where are they getting their food? How do they travel around? Who takes care of them? What other options might they have that they haven't considered, such as going back to school, making other work arrangements, or asking for accommodations at their current job?

This approach has enabled me to avoid viewing every person seeking public aid as a probable fraud, and even to steer some people away from applying for assistance that really wasn't meant for them, while still being able to help them sincerely and willingly. I've recently had conversations with several patients who are new immigrants in late middle age (somewhere between 55 and 70), who were asking me to exempt them from the citizenship exam to become American citizens, people a lot like Kee May (see Chapter 2). The exam is basic: correctly answer a certain percentage of 18 questions on American civics, be able to read, write, and speak some very rudimentary

English, and you are on your way to pledging allegiance to Old Glory at a baseball game that doesn't make any sense to you (my wife and her parents, Veterans' Stadium, Philadelphia, 1986).

"I can't remember anything," is the way these conversations invariably start. "I go to my citizenship classes, and I study, and I think I know, but then next day I don't remember anything. Can you help me with a paper, so I do not have to take the exam?"

Many of my patients in this boat really can't learn—they are beginning to show signs of dementia caused by multiple early strokes, or else have developed a pseudo-dementia (it's really a disease but not really dementia) due to post-traumatic stress, adjustment disorder from culture shock, or some other mental illness. Some are, in fact, in a downward spiral precisely because of their anxiety over the exam, becoming not only unable to learn but unable to function in daily life. They have heard about the angry interviewers, the ones who yell questions at confused people asking them if they are Communists, or terrorists, or deposed royalty, and they fear that someone will decide to send them back to the refugee camp, or worse, to the war zone.

I have an ever-expanding battery of tests I have learned to use to identify these folks, based on them not being able to think through how to get across the street or name at least eight different animals in a minute. But the ones whom I'm thinking of are mentally intact, just very nervous, and for the most part *have never, ever, gone to school for anything*. They were farmers in countries where school was not an option, or at least not an option for girls, so they never learned how to learn. And many, due to poorly treated chronic illnesses, torture, or the other privations that sent them here in the first place, are receiving disability benefits—which run out after seven years in the country, unless they have earned their US citizenship. The exam becomes the only thing that can preserve their modest livelihood.

Finally, instead of saying no and leaving the person dismayed and panicked, I started explaining myself. "Oh, no, I am not a mentally ill person, my brain is fine!" was one response. "I guess I just need a few months to study," was the reply from someone to whom I pointed out that, since he worked full time, he was not so disabled that he couldn't take the exam.

I tracked down a staff member at one of the agencies that teach the classes to see how they address the issue of older adults in the classroom for the first time. I had my friend who interprets many of these encounters for me start showing patients the cell-phone app that he used to study for his exam, so they could study at home in their own language, and connecting them with the interpreter who helps conduct the exam for those who can understand and remember the questions and answers in their native tongue, but not in English (a perfectly legal way to take the exam, it turns out).

The network of social services and supports is vast and complex; there is a reason it requires its own separate profession to navigate. Just as the social workers who work with me (and whom I treasure beyond rubies for all the times they have made miracles occur) do not presume to understand all of medicine, my colleagues and I are babes in the woods when it comes to understanding social programs. What exactly is an aging waiver? Who qualifies for ACCESS transportation? If we take the time to learn these things, and the sometimes convoluted processes for applying for the program, we can start to realize that the person who they thought was a fraud was just desperately applying for any program he could think of, or mistakenly applying for the wrong program—or knowingly bending the truth a little to try to keep from starving until something better comes along.

This is way more complicated than the panhandler rule, and that's as it should be. Our social programs, whether government-funded or private, are stretched thin, and failing to redirect someone who is looking in the wrong place, or call out someone who is flat-out cheating the system, takes precious funds away from people who need them, even as treating every person with suspicion demoralizes and insults them.

Maybe, we need a revised panhandler rule: don't just walk by and toss money in the cup, or refuse to toss money in the cup. Stop, look each one in the eye, and find out who they are. It is a lot harder to miss a person in true need, once you have a story—and a lot harder for someone who is lying to keep it up for that long. Most importantly, it is a lot harder for *you*, the one who holds the purse-strings, or the key to the magic gate, to forget that you are being asked to pass judgment on a human being, not just on a "case."

With the "revised panhandler rule" in mind, I want to come back to the issue of addiction. One of the great privileges of my career has been to work closely with a halfway house for people in recovery, usually their first six months after completing an initial rehab—or a short jail term. The privilege comes from the brutal honesty that a newly sober recovering addict has to employ, with themselves and everyone else, in order to maintain sobriety.

These encounters teach me about the lies an addict will tell themselves and the ones they have tried on the likes of me and my colleagues to feed their habit, the trauma they go through both during the period of active drug use and that which led them to drugs in the first place, and the seemingly insurmountable barriers to getting back to "normal" life after addiction. I've learned how much many of them despise their addictions, and how sick they are of living that way, especially as they age out of their "partying" years and begin to crave the stability that comes with not being a kid anymore.

I've also learned why the panhandler rule makes a good story, but the revised panhandler rule makes better medicine. At the end of one of my sessions at the house, I heard a familiar voice come into clinic—a voice that had been cursing me out the last time I had heard it. She had been clean for a while, but during a relapse came to me for pain medication, ostensibly to treat her for pain from a gallbladder removal that had happened over a month earlier. When I wouldn't oblige, she let me have an earful—loudly and threateningly enough that I needed to have her removed from the office. Today, though, she wasn't there to tell me how uncaring I was about her pain. She was there to say thank you, for standing my ground and helping her to see that she had, in fact, relapsed and wasn't just "treating a medical condition" by seeking out the drugs that had started her addiction in the first place. As far as she was concerned, I had saved her life.

Working with people in recovery, and really at a community health center in general, has also brought me in contact with a lot of people who have spent time in jail. A recent TED Talk by musician John Legend reminded viewers that prison is supposed to be about rehabilitation and redemption—and showcased spoken-word poetry from a then-current inmate at San Quentin Prison, who was due for his release in 18 months, a rare glimpse at the humanity corralled inside those walls.

I get that glimpse a lot in my work, talking with people in recovery, in halfway houses, and in transition. Often, I work with an organization called Aleph Institute, which specifically takes Jewish prisoners under its wing, shepherds them from their release into housing, employment—and my office, where they receive comprehensive medical care. If criminals and addicts seem to lose the human image in our eyes, then recovery programs, John Legend, and Aleph are engaged in giving the human image back to those who have lost it.

Within the past year my practice has taken up this challenge as well. It wasn't enough to have a "Just Say No" policy about narcotic pain medications. Sure, the patients weren't getting their fix from us, but they were still using. Seeing these patients as people with an illness, rather than as a nuisance, meant we had to come up with a way to help make them better. Thus was born our MAT (medication-assisted treatment) program, a highly structured program that uses the unusual opioid buprenorphine to help people transition from uncontrolled drug abuse to stable, functioning "normal" lives. The bedrock of the program is that we don't punish, we don't dismiss, and we don't scold. When people stumble and fall, by relapsing on narcotics or on other drugs, we pick them up, keep a closer watch on them for a while, and start back up the hill again. The approach isn't without its problems, but it creates an opportunity not unlike HAART for AIDS patients or immunotherapy for cancer: the chance for a deadly disease (yes, deadly—look up your local overdose statistics) to become a controlled, chronic illness.

The panhandler rule holds that the charlatans and scoundrels can't be allowed to take away our compassion. The revision holds that our compassion can't be allowed to blind us to the fact that there is more than one kind of suffering that people experience. Panhandlers, "drug seekers," and people working under the table while on disability are all trying to solve a problem that seems insoluble any other way. Communication is the key to entering into covenant and finding a better solution. The new rule reads, "I would rather waste my time hearing the story of a hundred con artists than turn a deaf ear to the needs of one person who is truly suffering."

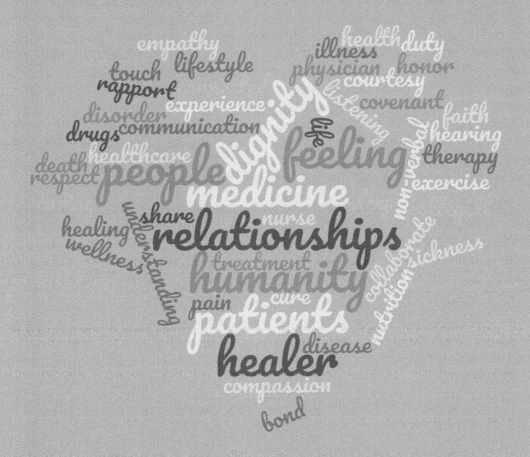

CHAPTER 9

No Time to Waste

It is said that even a stopped clock has the correct time twice a day. I think that may be true of the pace at which I see my patients, as well.

We're not talking about me as a resident, when my geriatrics attending gently told me I was, "among the slower of my colleagues." This is me, eight years in practice, spending most of every day wondering where the time has gone. The single biggest obstacle to doing an exceptional, humane job taking care of both the sick and the well is a lack of time. The time I have to make a diagnosis before someone's condition worsens. The time it takes someone to recover—very slowly—from a self-limiting illness. The seemingly eternal wait until someone can get an appointment to see me—and the longer-than-eternal wait for that person to get an appointment with the outside specialist to whom I have referred them. The time the *next* patient has spent in the waiting room and the exam room, twiddling his thumbs, while I have attended to the needs of the current patient. Why is it so hard to find that time?

My phone rings. It's one of the excellent nurses with whom I work. The team of them spend their days answering patient phone calls and performing the all-important function of triage. They're the ones who decide which patients need to be seen urgently, which need to be sent to the emergency department, which have simple questions or requests that can be met by phone, and which need to come in to the office to meet with another staff member.

"Dr. Weinkle, Mr. Roosevelt was just released from the hospital on Monday for pneumonia. He was told he must follow-up with his PCP within three to five days, and with the weekend coming, I'm really worried about him. Can we squeeze him in tomorrow?"

Of course we can; Mr. Roosevelt clearly needs to see me, so he doesn't end up back in the hospital.

"Do I have anything open?"

"Well, that's the problem …" I'm booked tomorrow every 15 minutes, and in one spot I'm double-booked. In fact, the official word on the street is that my next available appointment is three months from now. I am unable to "squeeze" Mr. Roosevelt in anywhere.

I'm also a pushover and a bleeding heart, so what I *actually* say is, "Put him in at 11:45; worse comes to worst, I'll skip lunch."

"You've already got people in your lunch hour and before the official start of clinic."

"Can one of the other providers see him?"

"They're full, too."

Go to medical school, and you'll never want for a job, they told me. People will always need you. Well, they were right, and there is not enough of me, or my colleagues, to go around. Doctors and the other professionals who play on our team are in demand—and my type of doctor, the primary care provider, the "family doctor," is especially in demand.

I practice in the same city where I studied and trained, so the students I now teach in my practice are from my *alma mater*. I've had some pretty outstanding students in that time (many of whom would make excellent family physicians, pediatricians, or internists), and I work with about 20 to 25 medical students a year. Yet, in one recent graduating class, a grand total of six students—out of a class of more than 140—chose a career in family medicine. Perhaps a dozen each chose internal medicine and pediatrics, and two took the combined medicine-pediatrics track on which I trained. That means only 30 out of 140 students have any chance of practicing primary care when they finish their training.

Out of 20 pediatric residents I graduated with, at least half of the class specialized, and even a larger proportion of the internal medicine residents, so it's more like 15 out of 140, or just over 10 percent. Nearly 90 percent of the newly minted doctors from that class will never practice primary care. The ones who do end up replacing a generation of their predecessors, who are choosing early retirement out of mounting burnout or frustration with the system.

They're closing their practices to new patients, narrowing their focus, eliminating care for Medicare and Medicaid patients, or leaving clinical medicine for research, industry, or administration. Meanwhile, the number of people needing primary care just keeps climbing. Babies are born every day. People immigrate every year. Modern medical miracles mean that children who would never have survived their childhood diseases now grow to adulthood with full lives—and complex medical needs that demand a medical home. The same miracles help ill adults recover and age, until they become seniors who need careful, thorough treatment from an experienced provider.

Large swaths of this population are serviced by a handful of family physicians, who "do it all," even minor surgeries. In reality, however, the percentages of family physicians who can really do all that are in the low teens, and family medicine residency programs have among the lowest "fill rates" of any specialty, even after non-US medical students are given the chance to fill the spots. Even growing the workforce by adding "physician extenders," nurse practitioners and physician assistants who in many cases function every inch as physicians, has not closed the gap—partially because the PA and NP students often make the same career choices as the physicians, leaving the same shortage areas as before. Attempts to grow the numbers of pediatric subspecialists by "fast-tracking" residents into critical shortage areas, like neurology and rheumatology, after only two years of residency can't overcome the fact that there are not enough pediatric residents to begin with. And every one of them who does specialize is one *less* primary pediatrician going into the workforce.

Why are people not flocking to do this job? Why do I feel like a member of an endangered species? Being entrusted to care for the diverse group of human beings that I care for is a gift that they give me. It's a chance to interact with the entire rich tapestry of human existence across the entire human lifespan, to hold adorable babies in the morning and frail, papery hands in the afternoon, to learn six different words for dizzy in the same day (my favorite: *kizungu-zungu*, in Kiswahili), to save a life before lunch and mourn the passing of one after. People will bring you cakes, send you cards and thank you notes, draw you pictures, and buy you shirts (I received a handmade suit from Nepal last year). Yet, given the chance to do this, medical professionals seem to be fleeing.

The reason there is so much demand for people to do this incredible job is partially because of the demands *of* the job. It's the most important kind of medicine. I think of a specialist as someone I call to bail me out in the minority of cases that go beyond my abilities to handle. I also think of myself as the person a patient starts with in order to figure out which specialist to go to in the first place, and the type of doctor that *everyone* needs to have when they get sick and to help keep them well. Furthermore, I am the doctor who keeps all the disparate pieces of a person's medical care tied together, the one who is supposed to make sense of all the pieces.

It's ennobling and overwhelming all at once. If we really want to provide care to a person, rather than a disease, and meet all the functions I just named, the following are some of the things we need to be doing: discussing end-of-life wishes, screening for depression, ensuring someone receives all of their health maintenance exams, carefully addressing medication side-effects, maintaining an updated problem list, and doing "teach-backs" to make sure we really were communicating with the patient, instead of just talking at them.

When we attempt to fulfill those functions, we fall hopelessly short. We're only providing slightly more than half of recommended care for chronic diseases or preventive purposes, whether we're talking about recommended "well-child" care or comprehensive treatment of diabetes. Every practice scrambles to increase rates of vaccinated three-year-olds, and improve the percentage of diabetics who also take a cholesterol medicine. Every practice fails. There simply isn't time.

It is of this situation that UCLA basketball coach John Wooden used to say, "Always be fast; never hurry." While I have had many patients complain about being kept waiting, I have never heard any of them gush about how punctual their doctors are or compliment me for being on time, except maybe sarcastically. They do, however, complain bitterly about doctors who they feel were rushed and didn't give them the time they deserved.

Conversely, they have only the highest praise for doctors they have seen whom they feel were thorough and committed to doggedly pursuing the best treatment for the patient, no matter how much time it took. Many patients value this enough that they even wave off my apologies, if I enter the room late. "Don't worry," they say, "I'm sure you were spending extra time with someone who needed it, and now it's my turn—so, get comfy."

Think for a minute, however, about all the things we do to cut corners in our personal lives because of being short on time. We buy our vegetables already cut up into the size we want them, because it takes too long to peel them and chop them. For that matter, we put our vegetables into a blender, so we can drink them because it takes too long to *chew* them. We put off needed maintenance on our houses, our cars, and our own health, because they are inconveniences that interrupt the flow of our day—until they become emergencies and bring everything to a screeching halt. We hesitate to start uncomfortable but critical conversations with our loved ones, because they cannot be rushed, and we simply don't have time to do them justice— but then we don't say anything at all, and resentment builds, confusion reigns, and misunderstanding takes over.

Even if we have the best of intentions, as my patients credit me with, the definition of "thorough" has ballooned over the years, making it increasingly difficult to find the median between thorough and efficient. In 2005, one of my residency mentors taught us that a "thorough" pediatrician would need 91 minutes per well-child visit to provide all of the AAP recommended guidance and preventive care for a seven-year-old child. Today, standard pediatric visits are 15 minutes long. An adult preventive visit averages 16 minutes in length, and occurs perhaps twice a year. I need to fit in a dizzying number of tasks. A primary care physician providing optimal care for a typically sized panel of patients would need to spend *in excess of* 92 hours a week working to complete that goal—more than twice what is usually considered "full time."

I see 15, perhaps 20 people a day, each of whom has 15 minutes of our time, but an entire world, an ongoing saga, which needs to be addressed. Today's crisis will always rise to the top of the list; the question is which other item it will bump to the bottom, or off the list altogether. Will it be the follow-up testing for diabetes? Will it be the careful review of medications to ensure that they are being taken, being taken properly, not being taken in harmful combinations, and not costing more than the patient can afford? Will it be the brief moment of eye contact and expression of understanding for the patient's recent loss of a parent, even though this isn't a "medical problem"—or at least not yet?

Then, there are the other patients not present that day, but who are part of my "panel." They may call in with new illnesses, old ailments, expired prescriptions, or disconnected electricity. Their cardiologist may wish to speak with me urgently—not because the patient is so urgently ill, but because they are even busier than I am.

I can easily get near a hundred individual patients entering my consciousness in a single day. To give an average of even 15 minutes to those hundred people would literally require more hours than there are in a day. Concede six hours of sleep and three for eating, grooming, and travel to and from my home, and now they get less than 10 minutes a piece. Oh, and don't feel sorry for *me*. I have colleagues who are pediatricians who have seen 65 *appointments* in one work day, without counting their calls and paperwork.

Imagine beginning each day of your career knowing that you were going to fall short of the standard of care *all* the time, by so much that if you were in high school, you'd be failing the course. If you devoted yourself to being thorough enough to actually succeed, you might actually have to time travel. Can you now see the allure of sitting in the dark looking at x-rays of the same body part on a screen all day?

There's something else pulling people away, though, keeping people from wanting to "get comfy" and have a good long chat with each patient. It's a truism that time is money—everywhere except in primary care.

A doctor goes to a cocktail party and is being stopped repeatedly by friends who ask him for off-the-cuff medical advice. Instead of enjoying the party, he feels like he's just having another long day at the office, except his patients are all drunken friends. Finally, exasperated, he grabs a friend who is a lawyer and pulls him into a corner.

"I can't relax; everyone keeps asking me medical questions! You're a professional. When someone asks you for legal advice at a party, what do you do?" asks the harried physician.

The lawyer smiles and has a ready answer. "Oh, that's easy. I listen, answer their question, check my watch, and the next day I send an itemized bill for my time. Word has gotten around and now almost no one bothers me!"

The doctor is overjoyed to have a solution to this problem—until he gets back to his office the next day and finds an e-mail from the lawyer with a bill attached for his advice.

Medicine is a profession, but medicine is also a business. Every profession is also the way that the professionals who practice it make a living. For all the buzz in print and electronic media over the last several years about how healthcare has become a business, or decrying the "medical-industrial complex," healthcare has really always been a business. Payment for services was expected, fees were set, arrangements were made for those who could not pay them—or in some cases, care was denied. These old-time practices did all sorts of creative accounting, collections-in-kind (cakes, chickens, you name it), and even intermingled financial records with their clinical records. They either kept the books balanced or had to take down their shingles.

What has changed is that a profession that historically involved a time-intensive, high-touch encounter between a solo physician and a patient, usually in the patient's home, has become a profession based on deploying a vast number of technological weapons. The bills used to be about the encounter, about the time spent picking the

Healing People, Not Patients

doctor's brain and unburdening the patient's soul in consultation; now they are about how much technology and technical skill was deployed.

A recent episode of leg pain sent me to the hospital for a Doppler ultrasound to make sure I didn't have a clot. I was legitimately worried; I have varicose veins, and had just spent 12 hours on a plane—coach—followed by 90 minutes on a train and five hours driving across Pennsylvania. When I woke up the next morning with a swollen foot and dull pain in my calf, I felt like I had stepped out of an internal medicine board exam. The bill came in two separate parts. After the "in-network discount," I paid several hundred dollars for the test itself, $20 for a "facility fee" (the cost of the privilege of having my test done in a hospital, or even a building owned by the hospital, and likely the source of the funds used to spruce up the lobby), and a far smaller amount for the physician fee—even though I never saw the doctor. His fee was for interpreting the results of the ultrasound on the computer screen. And, thank you for asking, I did not have a blood clot, so I suppose I paid a worthwhile sum for peace of mind.

Meanwhile, when I saw my own PCP a few months earlier for a physical, the total amount of the bill (pre-"discount") was about half of the amount I actually paid for the ultrasound. The physician's time in both cases is the *least*-expensive, least-valued part of the equation. The nursing education, social work support, and other services my health center provides, in addition to the doctor's services, don't get billed for at all much of the time.

I am forbidden from billing for a phone call that *I* initiate to a patient, even if that call ends up taking 25 minutes and cuts into my clinic schedule, or more likely, my dinner. I cannot charge for time spent writing letters to insurers, lawyers, government agencies, and the like—though they will reimburse my office for the cost of staff time and paper to photocopy records, as long as it doesn't exceed $27.

If I help a patient whom I am seeing with a problem that her child is having but the child is not present in the office, I cannot bill for that. And, if I run overtime with a patient I am billing for, I can increase the "complexity level" I have billed for, or bill based on time, if I document in explicit detail what we discussed, which then requires additional time to write the short novella required to "justify" the increased bill. However, the difference in compensation pales in comparison to what I would earn if, instead of discussing detailed dietary changes and exercises to help a patient with knee pain lose weight and rehabilitate the knee joint, I would simply inject some steroids into the knee in half the time and send him on his way.

Time in primary care is not money. Volume is money. Time spent with one person quickly reaches a point of diminishing returns; the same amount of time spent with multiple patients is far more valuable—to the physician. To the patient, every minute taken away from their visit by someone else's visit is further evidence that they are *not* fully human in the doctor's eyes—they are an RVU, a relative value unit, a number that means profit for the system. It actually creates an environment of pitting patients against one another. "I showed up on time—why does *she* get extra attention when *she* was late?" They are losing lifetime, missing work, maybe even risking termination, to be here—and someone else is using up *their* time.

This situation is the polar opposite of the kind of medicine we've been talking about practicing—but many of us feel we do not have a choice in the matter. Why leave medical school with $200,000 in debt and enter a specialty like pediatrics or family medicine, which are the two lowest paying specialties, and take a job where your debt burden is double your annual salary? Even if you were lucky enough to have a lower amount of debt (military scholarship, National Health Service Corps, California resident who got a spot in an in-state medical school), why choose the lowest paying field, when you are already starting your peak earning period anywhere from 7 to15 years later than your peers in high tech, and 4 to12 years later than your lawyer buddies?

Medicine may be a noble profession, but the people who practice it frequently graduate school with families already in progress, and the financial worries that go along with that. They are entering practice already with mortgages and children and thinking about how they can possibly afford to give their children the opportunity to choose higher education as they did. Even when doctors enter the lower-paying specialties, the pressure is strong to maximize revenue in some way.

Many physicians in this day and age end up employed, working for large health systems. Employed physicians often have "productivity bonuses," which are achieved by exceeding a certain number of Relative Value Units (RVUs), a unit of measurement of how much each visit or procedure is worth in reimbursements. The RVU scale is set by a committee at the Centers for Medicare and Medicaid Services and is composed of physicians from all the specialties. It leans heavily, however, in the direction of subspecialists and, therefore, tends to value the technical, rather than the cognitive, procedures. Even when the health system is a "not for profit"—a nebulous term—like a university, the model is universally one which aims to expand revenue, expand services, expand markets. It behaves, in short, like a business.

Private physicians "eat what they kill," to quote a crude expression that is used often in discussing business among docs. They earn whatever they get paid for the RVUs they produce, less overhead. For a specialist, like a surgeon or cardiologist, the answer is simple—cut more, cath more, earn more.

For primary care doctors, the answer is harder—either start doing more office-based procedures, even in cases where the indications might be fuzzy, or see more patients. The casualty of this approach is always the same: time spent with the individual patient. Every minute spent talking with one patient cuts into the ability to see another. Every minute lost from time with one patient cuts into the ability of that patient to tell their whole story—and the ability of the provider to deliver something approaching comprehensive care. That care is worth almost nothing, when measured in RVUs.

There have been doctors who perform unnecessary, and dangerous, procedures to pad their profits. There have been others who oversell the benefits of new, untested therapies and tests of questionable value and convince patients—and even hospitals and advocacy groups—that they are the gold standard and create a market for things that are not needed and not helpful. These people are a small minority. Most doctors are too ethical to knowingly defraud their patients. On the other hand, most of us engage in subtle behaviors that are driven by a system that pays its bills by volume instead of quality time.

A couple of times a week at least, a long-time patient will appear on my schedule for a "pre-operative clearance visit." They are having surgery (often, something simple, like a cataract removal or hernia repair) and are not allowed to have the surgery, unless I say they are well enough. Most of these visits, however, could have been done in the hospital, by an anesthesiologist who will already be seeing the patient that morning in the hospital, billing for the surgery, and speaking with the patient the morning of the surgery in any case, and don't require a visit with me.

Yet, when I'm booked solid, the patient will often be sent to a "pre-op clinic" at the same hospital to complete this visit, where the hospital employs primary care docs and mid-levels to see one after another of such patients, whom they've never met before, and bills for the service. For a long-standing patient I could have had a two-minute phone call or a 30-second email exchange with the surgeon to say, "Totally fine—clear for surgery."

Most of the folks coming in for these visits also arrive with prescriptions from the surgeon's office for blood tests. Both the blood testing and the visits themselves are meant to reassure the patient, the surgeon, and the anesthesiologist that they are being as cautious as possible with the patient. Yet, the national guidelines from the Anesthesiological Society of America tell me that most pre-op blood testing is of no predictive value regarding the outcome of the surgery or post-op complications.

We clearly need electrolytes on a patient with a history of chronic kidney failure, and a blood count on a patient with persistent anemia, but not on a well 50-year-old having a cataract repaired. These orders are not based on the patient's history—I'm the one taking the history, and they show up at my office already toting the "routine" orders. The order sheets they carry are pregenerated, standard order sets that don't involve any thinking about the patient, or even about the surgery being done. Since most of the patients receiving these will end up at the "pre-op testing center" for labs—and chest x-rays, and EKGs—as well, the system earns important revenue.

I am an unusual case. I'm not a part of either of our major health systems, and I'm willing to call the surgeon back to say, "Hey, Mark, you ordered some tests that are unnecessary, and I'm not going to run them." I do this, because when we test automatically, we end up with information that we don't want or need, and it causes harm to the patient.

The first type of harm is minimal, but still completely unnecessary: labs come back, and some minor indicator is outside the normal range. My favorite example is the BUN-to-creatinine ratio. In a patient who has elevated BUN or creatinine levels, meaning that their kidneys seem not to be functioning well, the ratio can help to distinguish a problem within the kidneys from a bladder obstruction or a lack of blood flow coming into the kidneys. In a healthy person, with normal BUN and creatinine levels, the ratio is meaningless—but often "abnormal," if the blood is drawn after an overnight fast, in a thin person whose creatinine levels are naturally lower, or under other random influences. Now that patients can often see their lab results before speaking to the physician, panic ensues, requiring a lengthy explanation from the PCP of why this "abnormal" value does not matter and cannot hurt them.

Worse, a non-clinician in the surgeon's office sees a result flagged as abnormal and puts the brakes on the surgery, requiring a detailed letter from the PCP explaining why it's still OK to operate, and sometimes delaying the surgery unnecessarily. Bad enough when it's a cataract, even worse when it is a painful condition, like a hernia or gallbladder removal, leaving the patient suffering longer than they had planned.

Sometimes, harm ensues when actual, but trivial, abnormalities are found: a low sodium level, a slightly low white blood cell count, unclear evidence of a urinary tract infection, a spot on a chest x-ray, or a "non-specific" abnormal waveform or rhythm on an EKG. Now, not only do we need to put off the surgery, but the patient also needs to go through more testing, some of it invasive, other parts of it involving high doses of radiation, such as a CT scan, in order to explain away the abnormalities. Not only do these tests bring in revenue, they also expose a patient to more harm. Any situation in which a patient ends up in the cardiac cath lab, meaning someone is puncturing his groin and inserting a long tube through his blood vessel into his heart, based on results of a stress test that they didn't need in the first place, is an unnecessary risk.

Sometimes, the testing is warranted—but there is still no reason to do it before the surgery. I recently had a patient whose hernia repair was delayed more than two months because of uncertainty about the condition of an abnormally shaped kidney that had been present for years, even though the risk for a complication in a hernia repair is minimal, even with the condition he has. The surgeon's office insisted he needed a kidney ultrasound before the surgery.

At that point, I called the surgeon to find out why this was all necessary to clear the patient for such a simple procedure. He almost audibly shrugged his shoulders. "Look, as far as I'm concerned, I would have taken him straight to surgery the same week I saw him; he'd have been home the same night and out of pain. I do whatever anesthesia insists on; when I operate at the other hospital, I do whatever they insist on there. It's all just stuff to cover themselves, as far as I'm concerned."

That's called waste—things we do in healthcare that don't add any value to the care we are delivering. They don't make the patient healthier, happier, or safer. They just waste resources—money, often, but also that scarcest resource of all, time. Waste in healthcare is part of a vicious cycle. It consumes unnecessary time. Much of the waste, however, comes from trying to *save* time by cutting a corner somewhere. Often,

Healing People, Not Patients

it comes from cutting corners in the one thing that ought to be the foundation of everything we do—communication, both with the patient and with each other.

I am still early enough in my career to vividly remember having to strategically plan out my trips to medical records to dictate discharge summaries on charts of patients who were already a week or more out of the hospital. With the changes in resident work hours, there is even more time pressure, made worse by the fact that the resident is often punished for staying in the hospital too long. Responsibilities haven't gone down proportionately to the amount of hours residents work—they just have to finish everything in less time. What usually suffers is anything not "directly related to patient care"—meaning to the immediate stabilization of the patient still in the hospital.

The old residency culture was different. They were called residents, remember, because they *resided in the hospital.* Even after that tradition ended, however, they were never far away. The pull to go home couldn't have been all that strong, if home was just upstairs, and the nurses knew where you slept. Besides, leaving the hospital meant you missed out on a good case, or had to leave the bedside of the patient you were really worried about. You could have that serious conversation with a patient nervous about their surgery the next day at 11:30 at night—since both of you were still awake. Furthermore, patients stayed in the hospital for a couple of weeks, so there was time to get med students in to re-interview them, examine them, do teaching rounds, and get to know the family members.

There was time for everything—except sleep. In trying to maximize time, residency programs ended up jeopardizing safety—both the residents', through auto accidents, and the patients', through medical errors caused by lack of sleep.

The culture changed as these hazards came to light. I trained after the work hour rules became national. I was mandated to work no more than 80 hours a week, whereas my partner who finished residency one year before I started frequently worked 110. I was once called into the residency office to explain a work-hour violation. I went back to speak with a family after sign-out and ended up being there for about 90 minutes. It put me up to 31 hours on duty, an hour past the 30 hour per shift limit. Only two years earlier, it would have been common for me to work 36 hours in a row or longer.

The message was clear. Get your talking done during the permitted duty hours, or get out of the hospital. Residents who spent too much time talking were labeled slow and often seen as needing extra help or being a drag on the team.

Even required communication, like dictating discharge summaries or even daily progress notes, had to wait until all the "important stuff" was done. "Calling a consult" stopped being a literal phrase meaning to pick up the phone and actually speak to the consultant, and referred to just entering an order that would pass from the computer to the clerk, who would call a receptionist at the consultant's office to "add that patient to the list." Furthermore, sign-outs, that hand-off of responsibility for patients between one doctor and another at change of shift, became more frequent, but less detailed, like the "elevator lobby sign-out" I described in Chapter 5. The car accidents and brain-dead med errors stopped—and a whole new category of errors, precipitated by doctors who were unfamiliar with their patients due to poor hand-offs, took their place.

In the absence of hospital-dwelling residents who never go home, hospitalist groups are fast becoming the norm in US hospitals for the majority of inpatients, enough so that many hospitals have reached a tipping point where a patient's primary care physician taking care of them in the hospital is an unusual circumstance. Private attendings round once a day, usually early in the morning before any of that day's work has been completed, see a barely wakeful patient, with no family present, and leave.

If progress is made during the day that means a patient can potentially go home, or to another facility. The patient sits until the next morning, ready to leave, but waiting on the doctor's orders—unless the physician who is gone for the day, can be reached by phone or fax in a timely fashion.

Residents used to be the "boots on the ground" who enabled private attendings to keep pace with hospitalists. As the work hour restrictions took hold, however, the private groups were no longer given resident coverage in order to keep the residents' patient load under its limit.

Hospitalist physicians keep things moving by being in the hospital all day, reviewing test results in real time, adjusting meds dose-to-dose, instead of day-to-day, and discharging within a couple hours of the patient being ready, instead of the next day. Research on hospitalist physicians centers primarily around whether they improve length-of-stay (meaning getting people out faster) to lessen demand for beds as much as it does on quality of care. It turns out that hospitalists do get it done faster. Unfortunately, they also have less time for "niceties," like phone calls.

Again, the culture has changed, and taken communication down with it. The busier the hospitalist groups get, and the residents that work with them, the less time there is for meaningful communication about the individual patients. I've been told flat out that there's simply not time for them to call me; sadly, they are not being lazy. Given how large the census is for some of the colleagues I have who practice hospital medicine, they are correct. Instead of a call, I get a discharge summary—a day or two after the patient has left the hospital, and all the decisions requiring my input and knowledge have already been made.

The first visit after the hospitalization, usually only 15 minutes long, of course, is spent trying to reconcile the brief paragraph of discharge narrative with the patient's impressions of what happened, merge two conflicting medication lists into one, and get back on the same page with the patient to try to prevent a return visit. A phone call the night of admission would have made the whole thing much easier. However, there was no time for the phone call, either.

Healing People, Not Patients

Continuing to follow one's own patients in the hospital doesn't help either. As I just said, the culture of private primary physicians rounding is falling by the wayside. So, what happens when one of the last holdouts has an admission, especially on the overnight shift?

"Jane, Mr. Roberts in 642 is having some abdominal pain, can you call his doc?"

"Sure, Barb. Who is it?"

"Some guy named Al Smith. Hey, Jeremy, ever heard of Al Smith?"

Jeremy is only halfway through passing meds to his eight patients for the night, because one of the other nurses called in sick, and the agency never sent a replacement, so he keeps right on working and doesn't look up as he answers, "Yeah, he's Jones' partner. But, he doesn't like to be disturbed after midnight."

Barb and Jane look at each other. Security has already been to the floor twice to deal with a patient in agitated delirium who was throwing (full) bedpans at them, and they can't really muster the strength for a grumpy doctor on the phone.

"Never mind, we'll call the overnight hospitalist."

Dr. Brown answers but is three admissions behind in the ER. "I'll send Dr. Shah up in a minute."

Shah arrives almost immediately, spends a few minutes with the patient and discovers, much to his surprise, that the man has a rock-hard abdomen and no bowel sounds, a likely surgical emergency. He sends the patient off to CT for a stat abdominal CT scan, which shows a perforated colon. The radiologist calls Shah with the results, who immediately gets the in-house surgeon to see the patient. The surgeon correctly assesses that the patient needs immediate surgery, accepts transfer of the patient onto his service, and whisks him away to the OR. Mr. Roberts is getting exceptional, timely care.

Dr. Smith is fast asleep. When he arrives at the hospital at 7:15 the next morning, Barb, Jane, Jeremy, and Dr. Shah have all gone home, and Mr. Roberts is noticeably absent from his room. Because Dr. Shah was immediately called away to "put out another fire," as soon as Mr. Roberts was wheels-up to the operating room, there is no note in the chart yet describing what happened, and no operative note, because he is still in surgery.

In this case, the cultural breakdown is on both ends—Smith for not wanting to be disturbed, and Shah for not seeing the communication as an equally critical step in the management of this crisis to the ordering of the scan or the consult to surgery. The nurses are complicit as well. Before the work-hour restrictions, back when my colleague tells me she ran over her pager with her car by accident—or at least, it was an accident the first time—nurses called residents with every change in a patient's status. Sometimes, they called even when there was no change, if the resident had been obnoxious the previous day. With the rise of the hospitalists, they have a "path of least resistance." If they are overworked with their nursing chores, they will only make one call, not two.

The problem with this culture change is that it causes problems for the other attendings. Dr. Chen doesn't mind being disturbed, and, in fact, she and Dr. Shah trained together in residency, so they know each other pretty well. Her patient Ms. Delgado is right down the hall from Mr. Roberts. Ms. Delgado's nurse, Steve, is recording vital signs from the 11:00 p.m. round, when he hears her start to shriek uncontrollably. Steve reacts immediately, grabs Shah, and hustles him down the hall. Shah spends a few minutes in the room, exits with her still screaming, barks an order for an IV sedative at Steve, and says, "She'll be fine; I've got to run."

Dr. Chen is still in bed, but not sleeping well at all; she's been worried about Ms. Delgado. She tries to get in early to see her but gets delayed, because one of her own kids is sick, and there is much coaxing and yelling to get the child up and dressed for school. Finally, she arrives at the hospital, but it is still after 7 a.m., and the shifts have changed. She finds Ms. Delgado in a stupor and unable to communicate with her—and notes that despite the fact that she had clearly ordered one, there is no translator phone in the room, and none of the nurses on day shift speak any Spanish.

It takes 20 minutes of detective work—more wasted time that wipes out any efficiency gained the night before—to figure out what happened overnight. The patient has received a fairly large dose of IV Haldol, which has knocked her out, and the order came from Shah. Chen angrily dials him on her mobile phone, knowing that if she waits any longer, he'll be asleep.

"Hey, haven't heard from you in a while!"

"Why did you knock out my patient last night and not tell me about it?"

"Oh, she's yours? Sorry, no time to call."

"Well, that's a shame, because had you called you would have known that she has pretty bad PTSD from something that happened in a hospital in Guatemala, and just needed to talk to someone to reorient, and maybe take a half a Klonopin by mouth, not a horse tranquilizer."

I understand Shah's predicament, though. Office or hospital, it doesn't matter—a phone call can potentially take as long as a whole patient encounter. The doctor might not pick up, and then I don't get to cross that task off my to-do list, or I might get an answering service and need to leave a message, then wait for them to call *me* back. I might be interrupting them and end up being an annoyance or distraction myself, breaking into a patient encounter or personal time, or sleep. I might start the conversation, only to get called away or diverted by an emergency, especially in the hospital, "urgent paperwork," an irate patient, or a question from a co-worker who didn't notice I was on the phone.

Healing People, Not Patients

The same could be said, however, of doing procedures—they can be messy, complicated, delay other patients, or get interrupted by other office business. The only difference between the procedure and the phone call is the RVU. One is our bread and butter, the other is flowers on the table—nice if you can get it, but not considered essential.

The decreased emphasis on communication leads to other problems within the system, too. Large studies have shown that doctors who communicate well with patients, who create the feeling in the exam room that they are on the patient's side, and who demonstrate compassion and caring for the patient's needs and concern, are less likely to be sued. The impetus to sue often comes from the patient's impression that the physician, or indeed the entire hospital system, doesn't care what happens to them. This even applies in cases where a clear error is made. Physicians who forthrightly apologize, when an error occurs, even if they are not personally admitting fault but simply saying, "I'm so sorry this happened to you," are less likely to be sued than ones who duck and cover behind the nearest hospital counsel.

Instead of building alliances with the patient, however, we retreat into a defensive posture. "Defensive medicine" refers to all the extra stuff we do to ensure that we won't get sued for not being thorough enough. Instead of spending lots of time with the patient getting to know them and understand their case thoroughly, we do every imaginable test to guard against every remote possibility of "missing something" that will get us sued.

The pre-op physicals I was talking about previously are a great example of defensive medicine—just like the surgeon said at the end of our call. Anesthesiology is among the most risk-averse specialties in medicine, and carries some of the highest premiums on their malpractice insurance. A mishap during surgery or afterward can not only ruin the patient's life, but the anesthesiologist's career along with it.

Anesthesia has responded to this danger by revamping their profession to resemble another one with lots of dials and displays to control: aviation. If there is a parameter the anesthesiologist can control to ensure safe "takeoff," "landing," and "cruising," they want that information before they taxi out onto the runway. If that means cancelling a surgery because the "weather" isn't favorable, they would prefer that to any risk— because an adverse event in the OR is as devastating as a plane crash.

Most of us practice in a far less controlled environment than anesthesiologists, and while our awake patients are able to give us more feedback when things aren't going well, we still run scared from the threat of malpractice suits. Being sued calls a doctor's entire worth as a professional into question. Every application for privileges, every license renewal, and every board certification is held up by the need to explain the circumstances of the suit. A stellar career can be marred forever by one complaint. The cost of the suit, as well as the increased insurance premiums that follow, can drive a private practitioner out of business entirely.

Clinicians who have been sued, even if they are eventually exonerated, often choose early retirements from clinical medicine, become depressed, or even commit suicide. Those that do continue to practice begin to second-guess themselves, ordering even more testing, in order to reassure themselves that they are not "missing anything." Furthermore, they are unable to do anything to relieve the stress from the suit, because they are usually under strict orders from counsel not to discuss the case with anyone. Everything stays bottled up inside.

After a suit, any ideal of the doctor-patient relationship we may have had to this point is lost. There's no covenant—there is only a suspicious, adversarial relationship. The "human being in pain" becomes another lawsuit in waiting. How can you focus on the patient's humanity, when you are fully expecting them to lawyer up at the first sign of error?

You behave like countries do when they are dealing with a belligerent enemy—by building up your defenses, covering all your bases to thwart an attack. In other words, by doing more tests, more imaging, and more procedures, since data, lots of data, is the best defense a doctor has. In court, you will be able to take the stand and say, "The mishap was completely unavoidable; we took every possible precaution and it happened anyway."

The fact that spending the time talking to the patient, and even apologizing when needed, might keep you out of court altogether is irrelevant. I learned that at the very beginning of my career. I shared my preference for openness in a problem-based learning group, at which point, one of my classmates flew back at me with the reply, "Well, you're going to have a pretty short career, then!"

Some hospital systems, like the Universities of Michigan and Kentucky, do encourage openness and apology, and claim to have realized savings of millions of dollars a year in lawsuits avoided. There is even legislation in some states to prevent a sincere apology from being used as evidence against the physician in court, in order to encourage more physicians to apologize. Most, though, still recommend a policy of complete disengagement; physicians are encouraged to respond to the discovery of an error not by notifying the patient, but by informing risk management (legal) and letting them handle everything. If a lawsuit is filed, they are not just discouraged from apologizing, they are expressly forbidden to do so by counsel. They seem to take the tack that my classmate was on—admit fault, and you are sunk.

Not only do the issues of waste and defensive medicine both negatively impact our relationships with patients by making us communicate less often and less openly, but they are directly intertwined. When we can't apologize, we're in a position of constantly defending our mistakes, saying they were unavoidable or inevitable. We are imperfect, and there's nothing we can do about it.

If there's nothing we can do about it, then we spend a lot of our time and resources fixing our mistakes. As such, I'm not talking about the communication mistakes that mean I waste an appointment. I'm talking about things like infected IV catheters, where "fixing the mistake" means several days in the ICU pumping someone full of antibiotics—and if the "repair" doesn't work, the patient can die. Even one infection is one too many, since line infections are completely preventable, if proper techniques are followed. But, if we never admit the error, the infections keep happening. For years a "line infection" was a clear and present danger in every ICU, and there was an expected rate of infections. No one ever dared to suggest that the expected rate should be zero, or that "standard practice" was actually causing the infections.

A few years ago, the Centers for Medicare and Medicaid services decided they had had enough. Patient safety organizations had demonstrated that "getting to zero" was possible. So, CMS decided to stop paying for admissions where line infections occurred, or reimbursing hospitals for care delivered to treat a line infection that they had caused through carelessness. They decided, basically, that a central line infection was healthcare waste—toxic waste.

Getting to this point required a process in medicine I can only describe as repentance. When we go to repent for an error, we take account of ourselves, not financially, but an "accounting of the soul." Was I in too much of a hurry? Was I too sure of my diagnosis, when there was room for doubt? Did I try to do a procedure for which I wasn't properly trained? Did I misinterpret something—or worse, simply miss something, failing to read the entire lab report or carefully review all the parts of the film? To ask these questions, we have to do something very basic, but very difficult, for most doctors—we have to admit that we are capable of making a mistake.

We are trained to be oracles on the mystery of the human body. Admitting that we can be wrong takes tremendous humility, something in which we are *not* trained. We actually have it beaten out of us. Morbidity and mortality conferences teach us that error is inexcusable, a cause for public shaming. The only way to own error is to admit that it happened and then immediately pin it on something beyond your control. Bad run of surgical outcomes? Well, what do you expect, you were taking cases that were so sick no one else would even touch them, so you should be thanked for the few cases that were successful, individuals who surely would have died in someone else's less capable hands.

Getting rid of the waste of fixing avoidable mistakes requires us to actually take ownership of the error, to admit that it was us, not someone or something determined to trip us up, that made the mistake, and that we are *making the same mistake over and over again because something is wrong with our systems*. Not by scapegoating the guy in the front of the room at M&M, but by collectively pounding our chests and saying, "We did this, all of us together."

Acknowledging to ourselves that we goofed is hard enough; looking someone in the eye who was harmed by our misstep, or facing the family of someone who died by some fault of ours is one of the hardest things we will ever have to do. It starts with a clean admission of error—not, "I'm sorry, but ..." or "I'm sorry; I was trying to ..." but just "I'm sorry." The injured party may want an explanation, but offering one in the same sentence as the apology is saying, "I'm not really sorry, because, as I'm explaining to you, it couldn't be helped, so it's not my fault." The explanation is not an excuse; it's answering the question, "What were you thinking?!?"

After the admission and explanation of the error, we enter the restitution phase of repentance. Ridiculously enough, healthcare has probably felt like this is something we were doing well all along—after all, when someone was harmed by a medical error, we were the ones that had to fix it! That's where all that waste of resources came from, isn't it?

Restitution isn't really being done, however, if someone has to *pay* for the repairs themselves, or through their insurance. Treating the catheter infection doesn't make up for Grandpa being in the hospital over Thanksgiving. And fixing the broken bone from when Aunt Gert fell in the hospital corridor doesn't really make her whole, if the hospital never apologizes for giving her the sleeping pill that made her hallucinate and wander the halls that night, off-balance and careening like she was drunk.

The malpractice system was actually created to ensure that "justice is served" for malpractice victims by obtaining payment for medical bills going forward, for pain and suffering, for lost wages, and for other hardship the patient and family suffered. On the other hand, an imposed settlement from a court, which the doctor pays grudgingly, doesn't represent repentance, especially if the doctor has never admitted guilt in the first place. We've already seen that the damage done to the doctor as a result can be so severe as to seem almost like a literal "eye for an eye" approach to justice. Add to that the resentment the doctor can feel toward the patient and the "ambulance chasing" malpractice attorneys, and the inability to repent can become pretty entrenched. Most patients would rather have a sincere, willing apology than an extracted pound of flesh in return for their suffering.

The final stage of repentance is to avoid repeating the error when we are in the same situation again. Some physicians respond to this idea, as we've discussed, through hyper-vigilance. "I'm sending you for a biopsy of this lymph node right away. Ordinarily, I wouldn't think anything of it, but the last time I thought that the person turned out to have lymphoma, so I'm not taking any chances!"

In fact, it is almost dogma among many physicians that "You always treat the last patient you had with this condition," even when the last patient's diagnosis doesn't fit the current patient's circumstances. For that matter, we tend to do this even in the absence of an error, developing habits that stem from a single case of clinical success. My mentor in pediatrics used to remind me a few times a year to always check the femoral pulses on physical exam, well past the age where this is usually done, because he once diagnosed a repeatedly overlooked case of coarctation of the aorta, a serious but rare malformation of the great blood vessels, in an 18-year-old boy by doing this on a routine exam.

It's actually pretty rare, though, that being obsessive about the particular clinical feature where the mistake was made will help us avoid error, or increase success in finding hidden diagnoses. Rather, it's fixing bad patterns. Have we been doing cursory, rubber-stamp physical exams? Have we been engaging in "premature closure" and settling on a diagnosis before accounting for all the loose ends? Have we been inconsistent in our approach to preventive care and thus missed a nascent colon cancer, so that the next mistake might be not a colon cancer but undiagnosed early glaucoma in someone who should have been referred for a routine eye exam? Have we just been failing to listen closely and value all of a patient's words, so that the off-hand comment about chest pain or about not wanting to get out of bed in the morning is ignored and leads to a death by heart attack or suicide?

Or, was there a systems error, where someone on our team failed to systematically read medication labels, check names on blood vials, or use sterile technique when placing a central venous catheter? These are the types of errors we need to learn to recognize, admit, and repair across the board. We must find the time.

Sooner, rather than later, there will be failures which are not errors, too. There are days that I spend in clinic where the "theme" of the day is "Medication Side Effect Day," or "Poor Recovery from Surgery Day." There are days when everyone is there for a second or third visit for a complaint that we thought we had addressed the first time, only to have the pharmacy not dispense a medication, a supposedly self-limiting illness fail to limit itself, or a specialist cancel a follow-up appointment that was supposed to provide all the answers. There are days when people who expected to survive find out they are dying. Death is not an error, as much as we might treat it as one. It is inevitable. Other human beings are fallible, and they are beyond our control, even if our missions are intertwined. It is inevitable that we will have to deal with these things.

When a patient reports disappointment, let that register for a second. Be professionally disappointed. Then, imagine the feeling when the disappointment is not a single outcome among two dozen that you will deal with that day, but *the* outcome, the only outcome that matters, and not just that day but forever. Now, you are truly sorry. So, say so. Because saying "sorry," and only "sorry," isn't just an admission of your own error—it is an expression of empathy.

You are not sorry because you necessarily made a mistake. Culpability doesn't matter. If someone else made the mistake, you are still sorry for the frustration the patient feels. Even if there was no mistake, and everything was done right, even if the operation was a success, but the patient didn't make it, you are sorry. Own the disappointment and sadness. When you share in the sorrow, you are earning the right to own the joy and triumph when something goes right.

Furthermore, when you don't own the mistake, or reduce the waste you create, or rein in your own excessive use of resources, someone else will inevitably take it upon themselves to make sure that you do.

About four years ago, a lovely woman I'd been seeing for years came through for a pre-op physical before having knee surgery, and handed me the usual lab orders. I know her surgeon very well, having done a little training with him in med school and moving in the same social circles, and I know he's a no-nonsense surgeon, who operates when he needs to and would never cut if he didn't think there was a point. Accordingly, I inferred that he also wouldn't order labs he didn't think he needed to avoid mayhem during or after the operation. This was before my favorite set of pre-operative testing guidelines was published, so I wasn't yet on my soapbox about this issue and went ahead with what he requested.

About three weeks later, and a week or two after the surgery, I was simultaneously hit with both an angry phone call from the patient and an angry fax from Quest Diagnostics. I had written my note for the visit for exactly what it was: a pre-operative clearance visit, ICD-9 diagnosis code V72.84 (don't write that down; the ICD-9 is now obsolete). I used that diagnosis code to order all of the labs, including a test of blood clotting function, which was on my orthopedic surgeon's list of what he was asking for—but which is now on the list of tests that the ASA says not to bother ordering, unless someone is on blood thinners or has liver failure.

Apparently, the patient's insurance felt the same way, because they got the bill from Quest and decided they were not going to pay it, because the test was unnecessary—except that it was already done, and the surgery was over. Quest, wanting their money, simultaneously contacted me to strongly suggest that I change the diagnosis code, and contacted the patient to suggest she pay up. Needless to say, she contacted me to suggest I do some things I won't repeat here, since I had gotten her stuck with an unreasonable three-figure bill for a test she didn't need.

Quest was kind enough to send me a very long list of alternative diagnoses that would explain why the patient needed this test. Sure enough, V72.84 wasn't on there—and among three pages of other options, not one described a condition from which this patient had ever suffered. I was stuck: I could throw up my hands and in so doing stick my patient with a bill that shouldn't be her responsibility, or I could basically fabricate a reason why I had needed the test. I was pretty sure it wasn't OK when it reached the level of insurance fraud, even to save my patient a couple hundred dollars. Several hours of phone calls ensued, monopolizing my time, the nurses' time, and the patient's time, until we finally found a code that satisfied everyone and unlocked the insurance company's vault—probably far more of a cost to the system in wages alone, than whatever the lab test cost.

Insurers don't just do this with pre-op testing, of course. They have medication formularies, with certain medications automatically requiring "prior authorization" to keep prescribers from overusing brand medications, when generics will do. They require pre-authorization for most advanced imaging, to prevent me from writing "MRI brain, with and without contrast. Diagnosis: headache" for everyone I see who is convinced that their migraines are a brain tumor.

They also limit the number of physical therapy sessions one patient can have in a year, to prevent repeated referrals to PT for every little pain, or to keep patients from treating PT like their routine exercise regimen. Some, like the military insurer TriCare and the Pennsylvania medical assistance provider Gateway Health Plan, require written referral forms for every visit to a provider other than a PCP, to prevent self-referrals and to force my colleagues and me to articulate why this other doctor's opinion is needed— and how soon.

Hospitals have fired back by creating Utilization Review departments—internally auditing physicians to see who over-orders and over-prescribes and stop them from doing so before the payers catch on. They have set up their own formulary committees, to limit the numbers of different drugs in the same class a hospital has to keep on hand, and to put a hospital pharmacist in between a doc wanting to order an expensive med (or an excessively broad-spectrum antibiotic) and the pills themselves. Ultimately, they create "pathways" meant to streamline care, which mandate certain treatments and restrict others, to bring care in line with some idea of "the way it's supposed to be"—whether that way is the most evidence-based, or just the most budget-friendly, varies from institution to institution.

The system works in a lot of cases. Indeed, it can be very hard to overprescribe, overtest, and overtreat when insurance and internal authorizations form the bureaucratic equivalent of the Great Wall of China between the doctor-patient dyad on one side and the treatment on the other side. There is a way around—but it's a long way ...

Aside from the additional wasted time these deterrents generate, however, they create another barrier between us and our patients. Rule-makers at the level of an insurer with half a million insured lives, or of CMS, that is responsible for tens of millions of Americans who have publicly funded insurance, can't possibly know that the patient I am seeing today has literally tried every non-narcotic pain medication on earth, except the very expensive one for which they don't want to pay. A person in a corner office downtown has not seen the family struggling to keep their oppositional-defiant daughter from smashing windows every evening, when they decide to deny the payment for her partial inpatient psych treatment. And, the robotic functionary on the phone (who is probably acting that way because they know that their supervisor will just overturn their decision anyway) doesn't know or care that the person for whom I just ordered an expensive MRI really does have weakness in their arm, which is one of the criteria to actually get the thing approved. They're going to say no anyway, because it's their job to cut waste.

Thanks to these waste-cutting measures, patients live with sub-optimal control of their pain, with the anxiety of an undiagnosed disorder, or without needed durable medical equipment, while their doctors, nurses, and social workers spend hours on the phone, over e-mail, online and on paper (because medicine still works with fax machines) arguing, begging, and pleading for the exception that proves the rule. I was always taught that if you hesitated to save a life, because you were dithering over whether you were breaking a rule, you were as guilty as if you had spilled the blood yourself. I can't imagine what my teachers would say about hesitating to save someone because of insurance red tape.

Meanwhile, the left hand giveth, and the right hand taketh away. The same organizations trying to rein in our wasteful spending on the one end are also trying to remedy the substandard care I talked about earlier. There are incentives for patients to complete needed primary care, enticing them to request cholesterol screening, mammograms, and annual physicals. Physicians can earn distinction, and sometimes even enhanced payment, for providing these services to a high enough percentage of patients.

On the other hand, if it wasn't documented, it never happened. As a result, we have to be sure to keep very careful—exhaustive—records. It's easy to see where the 91-minute well-child visit and the 92-hour work week came from.

You know what happens next. Women come in requesting their annual mammograms, when the USPSTF recommendations clearly recommend mammograms every two years. When I try to do the evidence-based right thing, they complain that I am costing them the $50 gift card that they have been offered as incentive, or the $200 reduction in their deductible.

I spend 30 minutes, some days, answering insurers' queries about why my diabetic patients are not on cholesterol medications—often on people who have such low cholesterol that they appear malnourished by that measure, or people who were diagnosed with diabetes two weeks ago and are still in denial about taking one medication, let alone one for a *separate* new disease. That, in turn, is 30 minutes I no longer have available to explain to that same patient why the cholesterol medicine is important. The insurance giveth, the insurance taketh away; cursed be the name of the insurance.

My libertarian friends will tell you this is the price of letting the government meddle in healthcare—bureaucrats trying to tell doctors what to do. Meanwhile, my liberal friends will tell you that this is the price of corporate greed—device and drug manufacturers driving up costs on one end, while big insurers attempt to pinch pennies on the other. They disagree completely on whose fault the problem is, but all agree on one thing: we are trying to heal, not push paper or follow cookbook protocols. Above all, we want to be allowed to be healers—and not be told by someone who never studied the craft, or who left it for some administrative job decades ago, how we should practice. We want our judgment to be respected, our advice to be heeded, and our time to be valued. We want to sit across from our patients, look them in the eye, and know that no one is going to disrupt our relationship.

When we don't get to do these things, it leads us to burnout. Burnout, as we remember, consists partially in treating the people we come in contact with as

---

impersonal objects. If *we* aren't allowed to be fully sovereign human beings, the people we care for will ultimately be less human as well.

On the other hand, that independent spirit can lead us to dehumanize people ourselves. Surgeons volunteer to do operations that are beyond them, whether because of the celebrity of the patient or because of the perceived nobility of the cause they are serving. Research physicians become so driven to recruit subjects for a study that they forget the needs of the human beings serving as those subjects—or so invested in a particular outcome that they let a trial go on too long despite obvious harm.

Any of us can have an operation succeed, but have the patient die, or cure the disease, while devastating the patient and bankrupting his family. Any of us can promise the world—and then fail to find the time or devote the attention to making it happen. Sometimes, it's hard for us to get our own egos out of the way of our relationships.

There's a book I recommend to some of my patients called *The 36-Hour Day*. It's about the impossible task of living a full adult life, while also taking care of another adult who can't care for themselves. I feel like my colleagues and I are living a 36-hour day of our own, trying to achieve the impossible feat of checking off all the boxes on the to-do list, while also having real relationships with our patients. Some of us solve the problem by simply electing not to do the relationship part—ceasing to be healers and becoming repairmen, or even gatekeepers for the multiple repairmen who fix all the parts.

I can't do that. Medicine is about healing body and soul together, about being driven to put myself out for people I really care about.

Excuse me while I find a way to add 12 more hours to the day.

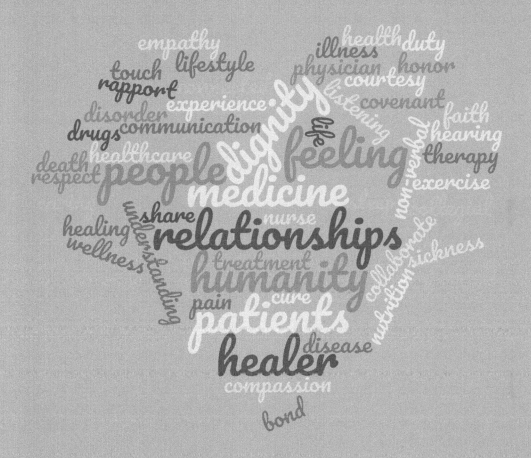

CHAPTER 10

Building a Sacred Profession

Reach your hands above your head for a minute. Easy, right?

Now, imagine that you are unable to do that, that each time you attempt to reach for something on a shelf above eye level, or wash your own hair, or put on a shirt, you are struck by a pain that makes you cry, "Aiii!" and that no amount of coaxing or convincing can get you to reach above shoulder level.

Then, imagine that the same pain, triggered by even gentle pressure, affects not only your shoulders but also your elbows, knees, and calf muscles, and even the chest muscles on both sides, in the exact location where you might feel the pain of a heart attack. Every time you try to lift something, or something presses against you, you are not only in pain, but struck with the fear that you might be dying.

You might try to go to bed, worn out from the pain, but at night you have the distinct feeling that you are on fire, mostly in the feet, but on a bad night, all over your body. My oldest son jokes about having someone spontaneously combust during a casual conversation, but this isn't funny; you actually feel like your skin is in flames. You're wracked by muscle cramps so severe that the calf muscles seem to be pulling themselves all the way around to the front of your legs. Furthermore, if you do fall asleep, it is like returning to early childhood, when you were still afraid of the dark—monsters under the bed, strange noises in the closet, and fitful dreams of danger, people trying to kill you or animals trying to consume you.

Trying to gain control over the disintegration of your body is tough, because you're beginning to feel like your mind is disintegrating, as well. Trying to learn a language, or understand the basic civics that will be crucial to securing your place in this new country, is impossible, because your memory has become like a sieve, with every new fact slipping through the holes in the mesh as soon as it's learned. You never went to school, but somehow back home, that didn't get in the way of living a normal life. Here it's an insurmountable disadvantage.

Not only haven't you learned; you don't know *how* to learn, or at least how to study. Even that wouldn't be so bad, however, if the parts of your brain that *were* educated, the ones that knew how to do real-life things, like cook, travel the neighborhood, or maintain a relationship with family members, weren't also beginning to fail you. You cannot boil a pot of tea without potentially setting the house on fire, because you didn't turn the burner off in time. You flooded the bathroom last week, forgetting to turn off the faucet in the tub. This morning you went out for a walk and couldn't figure out how to come home. When you finally did figure it out, you struggled mightily to open the door, until someone on the other side lifted the latch at last, to reveal that you had been trying to force open your neighbor's front door, instead of your own.

So, you've come to seek my help. You've waited weeks, maybe months, because I'm a busy man, and because the first few times you called, you found the phone system so overwhelming that you hung up in frustration and took a nap, resolving to try again tomorrow. Now, we have our time together.

Healing People, Not Patients

I'm on the other side of the door, about to enter. I'll have 15 minutes to sort through all of these problems you share with me, read the text of your aching body through my physical exam, and settle on a remedy. Then, you'll walk back out into a confusing world, hoping you can somehow successfully obtain that treatment, use it correctly, and be sustained by it for the next three months until our next quarter-hour audience.

I am in this profession to help people exactly like you. In fact, I spend much of my time with people who describe almost exactly the trials you are enduring. Dozens or even hundreds of people feeling their lives eroded by this syndrome for which medical science has neither a name nor an explanation. Yet, despite the similarities, each of you is unique.

I cannot assume that because I have met you, that the strikingly similar words I hear from the next person will tell a story with the same beginning and ending. I would like to be present and attentive to each of you, one after another after another, listening deeply, asking probing, but respectful, questions, and framing my words in a way that enlightens, heals, and uplifts. I would like to send you back out into a community that cares for you as much as I do, that will not put up roadblocks to you becoming well again, either by marginalizing you, undercutting my efforts, or placing me in a bind where my own self-interest is pitted against yours, instead of being aligned with it. But how? Let's take a time-out.

I've been a sports fan for a long time. Time-out is the chance to stop the clock, before it runs out on you, taking with it the last opportunity you have to change the outcome of the game. Time-out is the prerogative you have to get yourself in the right frame of mind, dust yourself off, and adjust your equipment, without getting thrown out at second base, or facing a 100-MPH fastball before you're really ready for it. Time-out is the saving grace when you are exhausted and the game is getting out of hand, a moment's relief to draw up the play that might turn the tide.

I've been a parent for 14 years. Time-out is what we do to children who are having trouble making good choices, a parking place on the steps or in the corner to calm down, breathe deeply, and remember what the right words were to say in that situation. Time-out is the thing that allows my youngest to compose himself enough to wipe away his tears and say, "I got my act together!" Time-out is the technique that my wife and I often impose on ourselves, when we feel ourselves becoming the parents we don't want to be. "Where's Abba going?" "He's putting himself in time-out, honey."

Medicine has discovered time-out recently, and for good reason.

Warren was screaming at me on the phone. I was off from clinic that day, in a meeting for one of the other projects in which I'm involved, but the staff in the office correctly decided that I was the only one who could talk him down. "I've been trying to tell you people for the last four years that the clip from my appendectomy has to come out! That's the reason I'm having all this pain. If you won't help me, then I'll find someone who will!"

I had been unable to crack the mystery of his abdominal pain. It was true Warren had a clip in his belly, and I had been working hard over the years to help him manage the pain, sometimes with doses of medication that made me wonder whether I was abetting an addiction. I was reluctant to send him for the additional surgery to remove it, since additional exploratory surgery in that area just usually causes things to stick together, and we had already asked one surgeon, who agreed with me that going back in was a terrible idea. As Warren's pain mounted, however, he was less interested in caution and more adamant—the thing had to come out.

That day he was calling me from the emergency room; he had gone there out of frustration with the pain, but still felt like he was being stonewalled. He was bellowing at the ER doc, and when that didn't work, he called my office. In the midst of my trying to calm him down enough to work out a plan, though, he stopped abruptly. I heard him move the phone away, speaking urgently with someone else in the background.

"Never mind," he eventually told me when he returned. "They're keeping me—maybe I'll finally get some help." Warren hung up, forcing me to call back to the ER to speak with his doctor. Apparently, he had developed a bowel obstruction—an inflammation in the area of his now-absent appendix was blocking off his intestines, and surgery might be needed to open it up. Warren went to the OR the very next day, and naturally, while they were at it, the surgeons removed the long-abandoned clip. Miraculously, Warren's adamant assertion turned out to be completely correct—his pain disappeared about a week after the second surgery.

Warren's appendectomy took place right at the beginning of the movement toward using the time-out in surgery. In a surgical time-out, the operating team stops everything they are doing to do some pretty basic stuff, so basic it seems almost idiotic. They stop before the operation to make sure they are operating on the correct patient, on the correct part of the body, on the correct side (left or right), and with the correct procedure. They stop after the surgery, but before closing the wound, to count the equipment and make sure that it, too, is on the correct side of the patient—the outside. For whatever reason, the time-out had not been carefully observed in Warren's appendectomy, which is often true in emergent surgeries like his. They were one clip short at closing time, but no one noticed—except Warren, every time his belly hurt him for the next four years. A time-out could have saved him a lot of suffering.

Leaving pieces of hardware inside patients is not good medicine. But neither is leaving poisonous words inside patients' souls—or leaving patients in limbo with their ailments, not knowing how or when they will ever feel better. Yet, we don't even think of these as being medical errors in the same way that we look at lost clips, hemostats, or sponges. We treat them as par for the course in our volume-overloaded healthcare system. But, all three kinds of mishaps happen for the same reason—rushing through the process of trying to deliver care.

Healing People, Not Patients

The difference between speed and hurrying in the John Wooden quote I mentioned in the last chapter is the feeling inside of being under pressure. The methodical surgeon doesn't feel like they're hurrying, but ends up moving quickly, because the movements are certain, elegant, and without hesitation. And like Wooden, they call well-placed time-outs, at the moments most prone to error, to make sure the plan is set.

The challenge in relational medicine, whether it's primary care, emergency medicine, subspecialty practice, or the hospital setting, is how to be methodical, when each patient and each conversation is a unique experience. How can I do the same thing in the same way every time, and end up with a brand new conversation?

By calling time-out. Each time, I am feeling swept along by the rush of the day. Each time I begin to sweat because of the pressure of waiting patients in other rooms, each time I recognize that something has gone sour in the interaction I am having, the situation calls for a time-out. The most basic time-out that I use is the equivalent of saying, "oops": recognizing a slip of the tongue, a clumsy move, or a poor beginning to an encounter and self-correcting in the moment. It makes me relish my visits with non-English-speaking patients, since I can pull myself out of a blunder by saying, "Chandra, please don't translate what I just said. Let me start over."

In the current digital age, we often function with mobile apps that show a tremendous capacity to learn as they go. Using Waze to navigate? If you drive through your own neighborhood by some idiosyncratic shortcut, Waze will quickly learn not to give you its standard suggestions for getting out of your own driveway. Learning Russian on DuoLingo? The app figures out what you already know, and naturally drills you extra times on the questions you got wrong, even remembering to show you how your skills from units you did weeks ago are starting to fade, if you don't do the "Strengthen Your Skills" units to refresh the bars. Listen to music on Pandora? Give the "thumbs down" to a few songs by the same artist and that artist will stop appearing in your playlist.

Time-outs enable us to do the same, but there is a special challenge to using them. Mobile apps have no ego; they are written to serve the users. Health professionals, on the other hand, are notoriously prideful, as we discussed in the last chapter. To be able to admit immediately to verbal error is a difficult task. Yet, it is what we do all the time in other realms of medicine, checking our work to avoid error. We put colorful carbon dioxide detectors on endotracheal tubes to make sure the tube has gone into the lungs (purple for "problem," yellow for "yes"). We double- and triple-check blood products before transfusing them to prevent an avoidable but fatal transfusion reaction. We obtain lab testing or get a second opinion to confirm a diagnosis we are 110 percent certain of—and often turn out to have been wrong and need to take ownership of that, too. We teach ourselves to say "oops" now, so we don't need to struggle with apologies for harm later.

When it comes to conversation, though, we need to be able to take account of our words and actions on the fly, while in the middle of doing the thing we are monitoring. This is where the skill of "listening with both ears" I spoke about earlier comes in handy—simultaneously attending to and processing the patient's words and our own, and taking note when we have said something we shouldn't have.

Sometimes, the pace of practice simply moves too fast, though. We need room for a time-out that really helps us "slow the game down," to be able to anticipate the difficult interactions, and to prepare ourselves for them, rather than dealing with everything reactively.

I've asked you to imagine yourself ill with the aforementioned syndrome I described. Now, imagine me, encountering a person with this illness in clinic, 15 minutes ticking off silently in my head. They begin by telling me of how dizzy they are all the time. They also have a headache. When that happens, they don't know anything, and want to go and be by themselves. I begin to formulate a reply, but they have already moved on to implore me to do something about the leg cramps. Just as I think I have come up with an elegant treatment for the ailment that they are detailing, they address their fear that they will fail the citizenship exam. I try to take a time-out, to pause and tell them how much my own head is spinning, but when I finish my reply, they simply resume their narrative from the very beginning.

I now try to take my time-out before the encounter starts. My clinic day typically involves four or five sagas running on parallel tracks: a systems issue with the vaccinations; two patients in distress at home, who may require urgent visits or referral to the ER; a pharmacy requesting prior authorization for a medicine; and a family asking for paperwork to be completed, so they can hire a caregiver for a frail elder. I also have to see patients.

On the back of each exam room door, there is a basket, and in that basket we place a clipboard with the "yellow sheet." If I'm lucky, the patient will have completed the yellow sheet before I arrive. If they have, they have written down for me three things they want to discuss, what medications they need refilled, when their last visit to the emergency room happened, and whether they are feeling depressed. I can take a 30-second time-out at the door in the hallway, purge the swirling worries about the patients *not* on the other side of that door, and formulate my questions for the person I am about to see.

The yellow sheet is a little like doing homework for a patient encounter, much like someone might do to prepare for a test in school, or for a meeting in the business world. Homework helps. I gave my first major presentation for other doctors when I was an intern, and ran 15 minutes long, so far overtime that I didn't get to part of my material and, therefore, essentially gave an incomplete presentation. I started rehearsing my talks the night before and, to no one's surprise, was hitting my time limits almost exactly from then on.

Doing homework on the yellow sheet, however, is a lot like cramming for the test during homeroom, or trying to put together the presentation on the morning commute. It is last minute and almost as rushed as entering the encounter unprepared. The better preparation is what takes place during the morning huddle (yes, I know, another sports term).

The huddle is supposed to be a hallmark of the patient-centered medical home, especially because it involves game planning for a patient's visit not just by the doctor, but by multiple members of the team. Nurses, students, medical assistants, social work, and occasionally even front desk or other logistics staff can participate in these morning pre-game conferences.

At one extreme, the huddle can easily deteriorate into a version of the "run-the-list" rounds or "card-flip" rounds some of the busier services in the hospital used to do when I was an intern. Trauma surgery was known for doing "thumb rounds"—thumbs up meant going home that day, thumbs down entailed staying until tomorrow. Next card. Rounds like this do nothing to create more meaningful encounters or highlight the humanity of the patient, though, and, as far as I'm concerned, might as well be skipped, if this is all they achieve.

A meaningful huddle does much more. I use my morning huddles to retell the patient's narrative to the team—a new medical student that hasn't met them yet, or a newly hired social worker who will be assisting with appointments, but doesn't know the person's background. Nursing will often fill in the gaps of what has been going on since the last physician encounter four months ago. Over that intervening time, the nursing staff may have heard from this patient a dozen times, and be able to detail their ER visits, medication changes, and conversations with home health workers.

Once a week, we huddle with the behavioral health team, who share what they know about breakups, bar fights, and suicide attempts, and work with us to plan what each of us will say and look for in our particular encounter, so that we are neither duplicating efforts nor missing something crucial. The medical assistants point out missing vaccines and overdue lab evaluations (a thyroid patient who hasn't had a level tested in two years, or a diabetic whose last recorded blood sugar was nine months ago). Front office staff alerts me to forms that need to be completed for delinquent light bills, school entry, work permits, and drivers licenses.

Huddling in the morning is an important frame shift for me. There are a lot of mornings when I come into the office and let out a little yelp when I see my schedule; I am scheduled every 15 minutes without a break until lunch, at which point, I have to both eat and transition to a remote site, or else a patient is scheduled during the lunch break. It is hard, in that moment, not to see each of those appointments on my schedule as a hurdle to be cleared in a sprint through the day.

The huddle is my chance to turn it into something else. It gives me the opportunity to remind myself of the amazing recovery from illness that turns the 10:15 patient into Mr. Frankheimer. It also gives me the chance to remember my promise to Mrs. Lama that I would remove the mole she was worried about, so I can review the procedure for a shave biopsy (it's been a minute since I've done one). It reminds me that at 11:30 there is a patient whom I've never met, but whom I promised to see as a favor to one of my favorite consultants, and who has a disease I do not know well that requires some reading.

In short, huddling turns my patients back into people, to repeat my "second sentence" out loud so I can remember what I love about them. At the same time, it also helps me to know what I don't know going into the day, instead of realizing I don't know it at minute 14 of a 15-minute encounter.

Huddling also helps to ground me within my team. It reminds me that I don't work in isolation—and how much additional work I'd need to do if I did. It highlights all of the things that each of the other members of the team, whatever roles they play, contribute to the care of the patient. Huddling keeps me humble, especially when my medical assistant (remember Radar?) finishes my instructions, remind me how old all of the babies are, and prompts me to order things I was about to overlook.

After a good huddle, I can walk into a room and say, "Ram, I'm so glad to see you. I heard you were in the hospital last week, and while you didn't have a heart attack, we're supposed to help you schedule a stress test and go over your medications to make sure you're not missing anything crucial. That sounds like a pretty heavy week. How are you today?" As such, Ram feels reassured, because he is coming in to find me prepared, hitting the ground running with moving his care forward.

The huddle is a rehearsal. Surgeons rehearse by tying suture knots and often spend the night before a major operation reviewing the surgery step by step. Docs who do procedures, like emergency physicians, anesthesiologists, or interventional radiologists, train on dummies, medical simulation hardware that allows them to feel what the intervention should feel like when it goes right—and when it goes wrong. One of the favorite courses in my medical school was the critical care medicine class, because we spent a couple hours of each day on the dummies, with a beloved professor who used to do things like deliberately unplugging the monitor or stepping on the oxygen tubing to see if we'd notice, so we could fix the problem.

Communication can go horribly wrong, as well, and needs to be rehearsed just as much. By practicing our words before we need to say them for real, and by resetting our "eyes on the prize" of meaningful communication with a human being in need, we set ourselves up to succeed, as we move into the part of our day in which we actually see live patients.

Time-out also happens at the end of a procedure—it's the time where we count our sponges. By the end of a patient encounter, I've usually mentioned 8 or 10 things I'm going to do for a complex patient—two or three medication changes, a referral or two, suggestions of dietary interventions, and probably a promise to look something up and complete a pile of forms. Without an end-of-visit time-out, I will likely leave several of these "sponges" lying not inside the patient, but abandoned on the exam room floor, forgotten and neglected until the next visit. At that time, the patient will ask me, "Hey, weren't you supposed to give me that emergency headache medicine, so I wouldn't need to go to the emergency department for an IV? Because you didn't, and I went to the emergency department for an IV."

This is the "what now?" stage of the encounter I discussed earlier. It's the stage where our actions tell the patient, regardless of the words we say, whether we are really with them, "coming to meet them," in between visits, or whether they are "out of sight, out of mind," until the next billable encounter. Can they call me whenever they have a question? Can they see me whenever they want a visit? Will I be watching to see when their results pop up?

We can't just address these concerns in the bracketed space of the exam room or the hospital ward, during the increasingly limited time we are allotted together. We need to do it in the spaces between. When a patient does not need to call back to get lab or test results, because I sought them out to tell them, I strengthen our relationship. When I reach out to a depressed patient after two weeks on Prozac to make sure they are not suicidal, I show them that I care, even when they aren't sitting in front of me. When I return the crucial pieces of paperwork without a reminder call, I let that person know I am looking out for them and won't let them fall through the cracks.

If waste happens because things we do to save time end up creating more work in the long run, then these extensions of the visit beforehand and afterward are investments of time that have the opposite effect. We expend time up front to save time, ours and the patient's, down the road, because of some crisis that will not happen, or some procedure that will be completed correctly on the first try instead of the seventh. It may be something as trivial as proactively printing and offering a driver's permit form to a 20-year-old patient I am seeing for the first time, rather than having them decide they need it the following week and take two buses back to my office to drop one off, which I then need to sign, except that I'm not there, so they need to come back a third time to pick it up. That's six extra hours of patient time, but the same amount of my time whether I do that work on the spot or wait until I'm asked. It may slow down my clinic day in the short run, but in the long run, I come out even, and the patient comes out way ahead.

Once again, the surgeons actually have something to teach us touchy-feely types. Anesthesia, critical care, and other disciplines that are heavy on procedures currently routinely use checklists to ensure nothing is missed. When I was a resident, we were piloting these checklists to make sure we used full sterile attire every time we inserted a central IV catheter in the ICU. It worked; the checklists were a major reason for the near-elimination of the central line infections I mentioned earlier. What would checklists look like for primary care?

The answer is that a lot of them already exist—and they are part of what drives those daunting statistics about 91-minute pediatric visits and 92-hour PCP workweeks. Furthermore, they drive me to distraction, thinking about how I could possibly reconcile

---

a regimented checklist like the ones we used in the ICU with having a conversation with a human being. On the other hand, how humane is it to say all the right things, and then fail to follow through on half of them because we dropped the ball? Ultimately, then, we do need to build such things into our practice. Our process for taking in a newly arrived refugee has come to include a specially designed set of lab orders, a state-sanctioned mental health screening that was developed in part at our practice, and proactive completion of school physicals, driver's permit forms, disability paperwork and TB testing.

At the same time, however, we have also held firm to making these visits more than just assembly line medicine. We allow 45 minutes for each person, even kids, in the hopes that we won't overlook a serious problem that would then smolder for two months in a person already trying to cope with moving to a foreign land. And nearly two years ago, we added a staff member whose responsibilities included developing a multilingual new-patient orientation program to explain our baffling healthcare "system" to newcomers.

We also have staff dedicated to making sure what I say out loud in a visit becomes a reality, instead of an empty promise. Of all the complaints that people have about today's medical system, perhaps the most damning criticism is the feeling of being abandoned—and the highest praise I hear is heaped on my colleagues who never abandon someone in their hour of need. While the medical profession may have fallen in the public estimation, the doctor who stands by a patient through thick and thin, who advocates for them and listens to them, who pushes them when they need a push, and who stands back when they need space, but is never far off, earns praise above all others.

This habit of thoroughness is one of medicine's oldest traditions, one that every generation of residents has learned from the one that came before, and from the seemingly omniscient attending physicians on whose shoulders they stood. A hundred years ago, it meant spending the night running back and forth between the bedside of a patient struggling to breathe because of pneumococcal pneumonia and the laboratory where the antiserum that might save their lives was being prepared. Fifty years ago, it meant racing to the room of the patient having symptoms of a heart attack to apply EKG leads, and then poring over the tracing with calipers to measure out the waveforms and decide how to proceed. Twenty years ago, it meant spending hours on the phone, ensuring that your patient got a place at the specialty clinic of your choosing, calling in favors from the specialist, if you needed to, in order to make the appointment happen.

Unfortunately, that habit was often instilled through means that seem almost military: sleep deprivation, social degradation, and public humiliation. Medical education was awash in maxims, like "The only reasons not to do a rectal exam are if you don't have a finger or the patient doesn't have a rectum." As such, the intern who presented a case to the team and didn't report the rectal exam was guaranteed that a senior resident or attending would bellow that line in his face. If the attending asked a question about the patient's lunch menu the day before admission, and the intern didn't know, the attending was likely to reply, "Don't know, or *didn't bother to ask?* Are you interested in being an internist, Dr. Slack, or would you perhaps prefer to transfer to the pathology residency, where you can't kill anyone through your negligence, because your patients will already be dead?"

The human-centered approach to medicine I'm talking about won't just materialize. It requires the development of new habits every bit as important as thoroughness: reflective listening, the curiosity to dig below the surface of a story, cultural competency, and tolerance (sometimes extended to people and things we find intolerable). These habits are not instinctive or intuitive; they will need to be taught. How do we teach them in a way that is not rote, not superficial—and not humiliating?

We want doctors who are humble, but not humiliated. The difference? Humility is the ability to say, "I don't know that; there are things I still need to learn. Someone else likely knows more about this than I do." Humiliation is the feeling that, "I don't know anything at all, and everyone knows that I don't. I would like to crawl under a rock and die."

Teaching a student humility means accepting an answer of, "I don't know," and telling them, "Why don't you go find out, and let me know tomorrow what you've learned." Humiliating a student is responding to an answer of, "I don't know" by waving that student off and saying, "Well, then, let's ask someone who *does* know something about this condition," and allowing the more senior or more obnoxious team member to show them up.

What we need to teach an integrated, human-centered approach to medicine, then, is a method that teaches students to know what they don't know, and pushes inquiry aimed at finding those things out—wherever and however they might learn those answers. Not just the answer to "What are the seven major causes of hypercoagulability?" but the answer to, "What is this betel nut stuff that all my patients are chewing, and why do they think it's a good idea?" Not just, "How do I secure a nasogastric tube in place, after I've verified placement?" but "How do I tactfully ask this woman's husband to leave the room, so I can discuss her gender identity and sexual orientation with her in private?"

When I was in training, the "soft" courses, the ones that taught these skills, were in the afternoon, when everyone was drifting off in a post-lunch coma. They were pass-fail, with no opportunity to earn honors, which took away any incentive to excel, or with honors to be achieved by doing some sort of "optional" assignment, meaning that anyone who wished to excel automatically stood out from the crowd as a glutton for punishment. Attendance was sometimes optional, and exams, the source of so much anxiety in our "serious" morning classes, were open notes/book.

Among the courses relegated to this academic back burner? Ethics, psychopathology, medicine and social issues, even epidemiology and critical reading of the literature. Morning was for learning the "real" stuff, like the Starling curve that determined how much stress the heart could take before quitting. Never mind that the afternoon courses would teach us about the stresses that everyone else's hearts were enduring, not just those with heart failure.

The one exception was our patient interviewing course, the most rigorous game of freeze improvisation I have ever played. We replayed the same patient interview 5 to 10 times per session, and each week changed our focus to a different thorny situation: life-threatening illness, domestic violence, sexual orientation, drug use, suicidality. It was the one time in my career where I can truly say that the attention to my tone of voice was as intense and withering as the grilling we would receive around the OR table in our surgery rotations.

Then, it ended. For the majority of students at the University of Pittsburgh and most other medical schools, this is the point at which their training in interpersonal skills screeches to a halt. This is what's called a "hidden curriculum"—just like the timing and the grading of the classes, the placement of all of these courses in the "pre-clinical" years suggests that, like biochemistry and gross anatomy, the information learned may be relevant in a sort of philosophical way to what we do, but the "real learning" is on the wards, where drug names crowd out biochemical reactions and a drive to be efficient, erudite, and highly effective crowds out the practice of spending time building relationships. The hidden curriculum teaches that the "touchy-feely" stuff doesn't matter.

My partners and I are lucky enough to train about two dozen students per year in our practice, so we get a bully pulpit to bring the hidden curriculum out of hiding. We put communication, compassion, and relationships front and center, and make sure the students are practicing these skills, not just hearing us preach about them.

We teach students to read—not literacy, but literature. They come to understand that our patients have stories, lives filled with struggle, triumph, defeat, and layers of meaning that are essential to being able to comprehend them and eventually help them. We can teach students to get their noses out of the "book" of hearing the story, and out of the "library" of the clinic or hospital, and experience what those lives are like.

The family medicine clerkship that sends over most of our students requires a home visit from each student—not a medical house call, but a social call, to see the environment in which the patient lives and understand how it shapes them, whether that is a Section 8 housing community brimming with new immigrants, an assisted living housing frail elders, or a distressed neighborhood where the student begins to see why the patient is afraid to go out for walks in the evening.

Our students don't just read about asthma; they read about the history of the Nepali exile from Bhutan and the effect of toxic stress on kids. They have a reading list that is culled from the bibliography of this book—starting with "The Second Sentence."

Not all students of medicine come from sheltered backgrounds or privileged circumstances. The so-called "allied" health professionals, meaning those other than medical doctors, often have a much stronger personal experience with poverty, hardship, and challenge than the doctors do, in large part because the cost and duration of medical school are a nearly insurmountable barrier for those coming from low-income families. Shorter, less expensive programs in nursing, physician assistant studies, rehab sciences, and pharmacy offer alternate routes into the healing arts.

We try to flatten the hierarchy, so that our MD students can learn to work with other professionals and to hear each other's voices. They rotate with the nurse practitioner and physician assistant providers in my practice, to ensure that they learn to see every colleague as a potential teacher, not just the ones with the same initials. They sit in on therapy sessions conducted by a licensed clinical social worker or diabetic teaching conducted by one of the registered nurses. They also usher their own patients through the post-visit portion of their time in the office, to see the work that is being done by the care management team, the medical assistants, and front office personnel.

But, we're one practice. The system, as a whole, needs to begin to treat these interpersonal skills as quantifiable learning objectives that can be taught, patiently and systematically, in the same focused manner that suturing, advanced life-saving, and reading x-rays can be taught. We need metrics that measure what we really want to measure. We need to employ a combination of existing methods to create a rigorous process of learning how to meet these metrics. Most crucially, we have to deploy those methods not just in a sheltered classroom environment in the sleepy afternoons of first year of medical or nursing school, but on the wards for upper-year students, during team rounds for residents and graduate nurses and pharmacists, in practice improvement projects for all levels of employees at primary care offices and specialty groups, and in incentivized continuing professional education programs and licensure renewals.

There are tools already out there to do just this. *Narrative medicine* is an entire field of study, and its techniques are already taught to students in a handful of schools. Students who understand how to treat a patient as a person and their story as a narrative, instead of a "case," can write notes and give presentations that don't just tell us about a disease process, but about a person with an illness. The interview can be restructured to include Arthur Kleinman's questions about the illness experience and its meaning, alongside the exhaustive lists of symptoms drawn up by Lawrence Weed. In addition, students can be trained to honor their patients when presenting by including Cole's "Second Sentence."

On the other hand, if ethical communication were as simple as adding a few questions to our interview or structuring our presentations differently, it would not cause us so much difficulty. There are endless ways for a conversation to go badly, and few people are born with the intuition to figure out what went wrong. The rest of us need a way of taking stock of difficult interactions and learning from them.

The Balint group is a structured conversation in which a treatment team, a group of students or residents, or some other collection of providers considers "difficult" cases together, not to "solve" them, but to clarify *why* they are difficult in the first place.

Psychoanalyst Michael Balint developed these groups to address the use of the doctor-patient relationship as a therapeutic tool, and to hone in on cases that were impacting the practitioner personally, through emotional responses, the investment of time, or the appearance of burnout. Studies on the groups have suggested that Balint participants may be better able to draw boundaries, recognize interpersonal dynamics and feelings that arise during an encounter, exhibit self-awareness as a person and as a professional, and interact differently, and more competently, in the physician-patient encounter.

I was introduced to Balint groups in my pediatric residency by two now-departed mentors, Bill Cohen and Ev Vogely. Bill ran the Down Syndrome Center of Western Pennsylvania, and Ev was an ED physician at Children's Hospital of Pittsburgh. They taught the 10 or so residents who came to that group at lunchtime to look into ourselves and figure out *why* certain cases were bothering us, to understand how we had gotten to the point of frustration with these specific children and their families.

It was over lunch, in that basement conference room, that I first recognized that when I encountered families that wouldn't vaccinate their children, I immediately felt a self-righteous anger well up inside me, one that I could not control, once I allowed it to surface. It wasn't my day to present; a fellow resident was fuming about a situation of this type that he had dealt with in *his* resident clinic. I felt myself cheering him on, silently.

Bill Cohen, who, besides his extensive collection of Grover ties, I remember most for his compassion not just for his tiny and vulnerable patients but for generations of vulnerable learners, never blinked. Instead, he calmly, patiently, drew out my friend with one gentle question at a time, gradually bringing down the pitch of his voice and expanding his insight into what had made him angry in the first place.

When that exchange was over, Ev Vogely took over with a story of her own. Several years earlier, she had cared for an unvaccinated school-aged child with cough and difficulty breathing during an outbreak of whooping cough (pertussis). After determining that this child did *not* have whooping cough, she implored the family, with an extensive data dump on the risks of the disease, to reconsider their stance on vaccines. "And do you know what they did?" she asked us. "They turned to the child and said, in a sing-song, mocking tone, 'This is what doctors do—they try to scare you.'" The session, as a whole, taught me not to expect myself to suddenly know the right thing to say in every situation, and not to expect that I would somehow "outgrow" my emotional responses as a more senior clinician—only that I would be better able to recognize what was going on.

The insight of that day has taken 10 years to finally sink in, but it is a perfect example of how training medical professionals to recognize their emotions and where they come from leads to better communication.

The "alternative medicine" community is booming, with countless modalities of treatment available. These alternatives range from the venerable, such as acupuncture, traditional Chinese herbal medicine, to the newer modalities of chiropractic and osteopathy, and include both well-tested approaches and sheer quackery. Mainstream healers cannot help but encounter patients who have espoused one or more of the alternative ideas, be it taking large amounts of vitamin supplements, yet refusing to take any prescription pharmaceuticals, engaging in colonic purges, nutritionally suspect fasts, or other hazardous practices, adopting incredibly restrictive diets requiring mega doses of hard-to-get foods, or opting for alternative screening and imaging practices, instead of the standard preventive medicine approach.

The conflict this creates drives many physicians crazy. When discussing the use of the white coat in Chapter 5, I alluded to the tarnished reputation of the medical profession in the 21st century. Many who are enthusiasts of alternative medicine espouse that party line, namely that doctors hide things from their patients, are completely corrupted by industry, or perhaps don't really know what they are talking about in the first place, and the savvy patient who does a little research, or reads a book on the subject (usually written by a doctor who thinks their colleagues aren't as smart as they are) can outsmart the doctor.

In my own experience, this happens a lot with thyroid disease, menopause, and other issues related to hormonal imbalance. Patients come in for consultation, describing a wide variety of symptoms, which through independent research they have decided must be due to one of these imbalances. When my testing does not reveal any abnormality, or when my clinical judgment (meaning my opinion formed by listening to the story and the patient's body during physical exam, without benefit of blood tests) suggests that the symptoms actually point to a different diagnosis, the patient often produces a whole set of labs from an outside lab (usually a proprietary one), repeating the same tests I have done, or perhaps others I have heard of which are not validated clinically, with a whole list of things circled as abnormal, often at values which are solidly normal, according to any measure I've ever seen. "I know you don't believe me, doc, but these labs show otherwise, and my chiropractor/naturopath/acupuncturist said I should come to you for this prescription," they reply, handing me a prescription blank already written out for them, but waiting for my signature. I know colleagues who feel almost as if their patients are being unfaithful to them in this situation. "If you don't trust my judgment," they protest, "Why bother seeing me?"

None of the anti-establishment ideas raises as much ire as the anti-vaccine movement. That welling anger I first recognized sitting in my Balint group in residency stems from the fact that vaccines are the treatment in which I feel most confident—if they don't trust my judgment on vaccines, what will they believe? It bubbles up more when I think about vaccines being one of two factors (the other is closed sewer systems) that account for 90 percent of the twentieth century gains in life expectancy in the US.

It begins to spill over when I realize that the pre-market testing for vaccines is often significantly more rigorous than for most of the medicines I prescribe, while the "science" most often quoted to criticize vaccines originated in a single, fraudulent study of 12 subjects, conducted by a man who has since been stripped of his license to practice medicine in the UK. It finally erupts, when I remember that the man who refused cholesterol medicine may have a heart attack that will kill him and devastate his family, but the woman who refused to vaccinate her child may be creating the point of entry for a pertussis outbreak that will ravage the whole community. I don't even come close to the anger of some of my colleagues, who will dismiss a family from their practice if their child isn't on the normal vaccine schedule by four to six months of age.

It took the skills I learned in Balint, and the humility to recognize my own failures, to realize that never once did I "convert" a family by railing about vaccines in our visits. If anything, my tone and my self-righteousness made them dig in their heels. The visits would take an hour apiece, even for an entirely well child. I would leave exhausted, demoralized, and unable to do much good for the next person I saw, who had already been waiting 45 minutes to see a doctor, who was nearly useless to them.

One day, I just stopped. I unpacked the conversations bit by bit, until I could spell out the process I described in the last paragraph, the progression of negative emotion that took place inside me each time someone said, "Oh, we've decided not to vaccinate."

Once I recognized this, my tone changed. I heard the stories people told me, the sources they presented, the arguments they made in favor of their decisions. I didn't change my mind; I still believe firmly in the worth of vaccinating. But, I changed my approach. I honored their stories, provided my own stories and arguments, and always ended by saying, "I'm really sorry you're choosing this approach; I know how much we both love Katrina, and I would hate for you to miss this opportunity to protect her against disease. I hope the next time we talk you'll think differently." They sign a refusal form, we move on to other topics, and we salvage a lot of common ground. The visits take 18 to 20 minutes, and I leave thinking about the cute baby, not what an idiot I made of myself.

In 2015, an unvaccinated teenager brought measles to Disneyland, and something remarkable happened. I began to see a trickle of families with whom I had held serious, but *calm*, conversations about vaccination, who two or three years earlier had left the office with their children completely unprotected, returning to see me, having changed their minds. They didn't come back because I browbeat them into coming in. They came because I held a respectful conversation with them and then left the decision to them; when circumstances around them made them wonder if perhaps I was right after all, they sought care.

It hasn't worked for everyone, and that's part of the lesson: there are no magic bullets in conversation, just like no surgery and no pill works for everyone. In those conversations, however, where I had taken time to see an individual parent, instead of just another "anti-vaxxer," I had been able to find something that resonated with the *person*, something that finally bore fruit two years later.

The hardest part of getting to that point was that rehearsing the conversations I needed to have with these families had to happen in real time, in real patient opportunities. Cynical patients often joke that they don't like it when we refer to "practicing medicine"—they want us to treat them when we already know what we're doing. In this case, they're right—we are practicing our conversation skills on them, test-driving them while we're actually seeing patients. Every day, I try to correct something I know I said awkwardly the day before—and sometimes I succeed only in coming up with another awkward thing I'll need to correct the next day.

Medicine is full of challenging conversations. My residency had a communication workshop built in every year for the purpose of rehearsing conversations about everything from addiction to abusive relationships to error and apology. It was groundbreaking—but inadequate. The training itself was great. In fact, one of the leaders of the workshop is a national pioneer in teaching conversation, through a program called Oncotalk, which trains providers how to speak to cancer patients about death.

It was inadequate, however, because it happened every year, for a single day. We were learning for 364 days to prescribe antibiotics, diagnose thyroid disease, and stabilize patients in acute heart failure. We studied how to talk to people for one day. You do the math.

We need more practice than that, and practice that doesn't happen on live patients during their all-too-brief visits. I've started working conversation practice into my huddles, asking students how they think they might approach a tough conversation I anticipate having with the patient that day, or asking my colleagues around the room for suggestions. We precept these conversations, too. A student might come out of a room saying, "I get the impression Mr. Harding thinks he's dying, but I don't know if he's ready to accept it," I will come back with, "What could you ask to help tease that out—and what will you say if he says, 'Yes?'"

But, like the yellow-sheet time-out, this is like cramming for an exam on the bus. We already know which conversations are going to be hard; why not practice them in advance, to get really good at saying really hard stuff?

Unfortunately, the kind of simulators that they used for the critical care course I talked about from my med school days don't do "meaningful conversation," any more than IBM's Watson computer is ready to write songs with Bob Dylan. Furthermore, human "simulators," like patient actors, are hard to come by, with a significant cost attached to training and hiring them. The interviewing class at my medical school often brought me into close quarters with actors I had just seen on stage in a local professional theater production the week before—patient simulation turned out to be a better day-job than waiting tables.

One of the key justifications for the expense of the current USMLE Step 2 Clinical Skills Exam, and other iterations of the "OSCE" exam, is that it requires large numbers of such actors. By contrast, a patient simulation machine may cost thousands or even tens of thousands of dollars up front, plus maintenance, but it doesn't get paid by the hour and can be in almost continuous use, even allowing for nighttime use during overnight shifts. It's just that the type of machine we need hasn't been invented yet.

Yet, there is potential for technology to help. A recent video game called, "That Dragon, Cancer," intends to take the player deep enough into the world of a young boy dying of brain cancer that they experience the emotions of the characters in the game. Scenes in the game depict the doctor discussing MRI findings with the family and the nurse lauding her institution's palliative care capabilities—and might just provide professionals playing the game with a window on how well, or poorly, they themselves would handle the same task.

Firsthand experience tells me how easily one can be "sucked in" to the world of a far less-intense video game (anyone want to waste excessive time playing "Bejeweled" with me?). Character-driven games, like "The Sims," or the "make your own high-school recruit" version of Electronic Arts' NCAA football game (my sons' favorite) can keep attention riveted far better than the most realistic "sit-back" movie or TV show, because they present challenges for the player to solve and reward the solution in a dopamine-releasing way that keeps people coming back. Could this neurotransmitter-mediated magic be harnessed to teach communication?

Until we figure out how, our colleagues and our patients remain the best study guides we have. Whether we just flat out admit to our patients that we are trying to buff up our communication skills and ask for feedback at the end of the encounter, or debrief with our colleagues over lunch, we just need to put communication on the agenda. We think nothing of calling a "curbside" consult to see if we prescribed the right medication for a tropical infection we don't see very often.

We need to start checking ourselves just as routinely on the words we use and the quality of our listening, calling "curbside" consults with our psychologists, palliative care consultants, or family doctors ("Hey Jim, it's Seema. Listen, your guy's heart failure is totally treatable, but he's really resistant to the idea of medication. If you were having this discussion, instead of me, how would you negotiate this with him?") on what to say, how to say it, and what to keep to ourselves. We also need to admit that it is easier, not harder, to talk to our patients when they are activated and advocating well for themselves—to encourage, rather than fear, the practice of reading books on "how to talk to your doctor so they listen" or frequenting websites that educate patients on the diseases they're worried about.

Our students play a role, too. Med students have always been relied on to gather information, because for better or worse, they take the most thorough histories, usually because they do not have the confidence to decide to skip over something, so they ask *every* question they can think of. When it comes to improving communication and getting a complete picture of a person, assignments like the home visit I described previously, or a health literacy interview they are assigned to do during the same month, can provide tremendous insight, not only for the developing student, but for me taking care of the patient. "I don't think Mr. Jones really understood your instructions about his insulin. Can you come back in the room and re-teach that?" Or, "You'll never believe what I learned about Mrs. Mukembe yesterday at the home visit—her whole story suddenly makes so much more sense. If only we had asked about how her family made a living in the CAR, we'd have uncovered this two weeks ago."

It will require humility to hear this from our students—yet no more so than to hear, "I looked up the most recent Cochrane review on aspirin use in well-controlled diabetics—it really *doesn't* look like it provides any benefit. Do you want me to call Mr. Applegate to tell him 'never mind the aspirin,' or do you want to do it?"

Students have a lot to teach us about relationships. I remember a student I had on the wards as a resident, who in fact had quite a lot to learn about professionalism regarding her attitudes toward her colleagues and her work. But, when it came to sustaining a relationship with a patient, she was remarkable.

In parallel to the patients she followed on our internal medicine service, she would check in each day to the pediatric record to follow-up on her patient, a young boy, from the previous month. She frequently took the five-minute walk through the bridge that connected the two hospitals to visit him, and checked in with his family, after he was finally discharged. This kind of behavior conveys real caring and investment, "ownership" of her responsibility to this child, and seems to emanate naturally from many students, though certainly not all.

There are mid-career attendings who have this same gift, but they are rare indeed. Students usually have a "census" of just a few patients on hospital rotations, sometimes just one or two a month, depending on the number of other students, "turnover" of patients, and season of the year. My most enterprising family medicine students, who step up for every patient encounter they can, and keep running lists of who they've seen, may end up seeing as many as 80 unique patients a month, but that volume is not repeated from month to month, and their involvement with many of the patients is tangential. My own "census" or "panel" of patients numbers in the thousands, even after excluding "inactive" patients who have moved away or changed doctors.

Yet, I worry about, wonder about, and check up on some of my patients routinely. They are grateful and often flattered at the attention, but it pains me to think that I am somehow favoring, cherry-picking, or simply choosing at random who remains in my active attention and who does not. How am I supposed to decide fairly who needs the extra TLC?

Patient-centered medical home practices keep registries of patients with certain conditions, but these almost always center around targeted conditions, such as diabetes or vaccination rates, and have numeric values that trigger the medical home to "go out seeking" the patient: a lab value that crosses an unacceptable threshold, or a null value in a box that tells whether or not a child has had a measles vaccine. If the statistics lie, or a patient has a condition, including a social circumstance, that isn't on the tracking list, then they fly under the radar.

We might complain about how much record-keeping the PCMH designation requires, but the fact is, we're only tracking a handful of conditions or markers at one time. What about the rest of the countless problems facing our patients? I've often thought of keeping a "worry list" in my desk of people I felt like needed closer follow-up. A nurse I worked with once described it as her little private island, where she would put all the people who needed extra protection in life.

But, what would the criterion be for "voting someone onto the island," or putting them on the list? Pity? A visceral reaction of concern? Doesn't that still leave plenty of room for error, for leaving out those people that, for one of the reasons we've discussed, don't evoke the same level of empathy as the others?

There's a process underway that might help, though it's very much a reactive process. Anytime my partners and I are notified of an emergency room visit by one of our patients, we try to identify if it was avoidable, or unavoidable. For the first few months, it seemed awfully judgmental—who were we to say if it was "not a real emergency?" Like Marty in Chapter 4, I'm certain most of the patients would tell me, "It sure *felt* like an emergency at the time!"

But, we were looking for things we—or anyone—could have done so that the problem didn't need to be resolved in the most expensive, least patient-centered part of our medical system. Were there barriers to reaching the on-call doctor, like not being able to understand the phone message due to language? A mistaken understanding of what the ER, as opposed to the urgent care or the PCP office, was for? Or, frustration at not being able to get a timely appointment in the office, which led the patient to assume it was the ER, or waiting three more weeks?

We are now in the second phase, where we reach out to each patient to set up the appropriate follow-up, and to ask the question, "Why? What could we have done that might have made it unnecessary for you to go to the ER?" Maybe, they didn't get the meds we called in and felt worse. Maybe, they are being abused and it finally reached the point where there was an injury that could not be hidden with clothes and makeup. Whatever the reason, we are building a learning system, one that both reaches out to the patients to better care for what is troubling them, and one that self-corrects by identifying problems the morning after they happen, not months or years later.

The next phase, I think, is to anticipate these morning ER mop-up huddles, when the patients are still in the office, or at any point when a worry warning goes off in our heads. Maybe, an end-of-the-day huddle, like a bookend to the morning huddle, could identify potentially vulnerable patients with a single question: "What are the potential issues that could cause bad outcomes in this patient before the next time we meet, and how can I or someone else on the team intervene to prevent that outcome?"

Healing People, Not Patients

Maybe, the actual patient visits could conclude with the questions, "When should we see each other next, and what kind of communication do we need to have in between? What are we both worried about that we need to plan for?" It would close the visit the same way it opened—with setting an agenda. Instead of paternalistically placing someone on a "worry list" or imagining them on a magically protected "island," we can partner to ensure a better outcome through a more active relationship.

Of course, we can do all of this, and it will amount to spitting in a hurricane. What good is a medical home, if the medical neighborhood around it is collapsing?

About nine years ago, I went to a breakfast meeting with Ruth Messinger, who at the time was the head of the charity American Jewish World Service. AJWS is a fascinating charity, because it handles giving and world-repair in much the same way that I've suggested approaching medicine—collaboratively, seeing the people it is aiding as partners, rather than helpless victims, and targeting its efforts, based on what home-grown activists are already doing to respond to disasters, combat discrimination, or alleviate poverty.

I was in my last year of residency at the time and itching to do something charitable, to go beyond the basic struggle to keep up with demands that defines most residents' lives. I knew AJWS ran study and volunteer trips around the world, to Vietnam and Mozambique and Peru, for as few as 10 days and as long as six months. But, there was one thing they didn't seem to do.

"Ruth," I asked, when the question period came around, "I'm a medical resident. Would AJWS ever consider a medical mission trip?"

"Of course not," she responded immediately, with such finality that I thought it was all the response she was going to give.

"Listen," she continued after a deliberate pause to let that sink in, "there are hundreds of organizations that do that. They recruit surgeons or family docs or optometrists, drop them somewhere for a couple weeks, and watch people line up. They deliver care that is so far advanced beyond anything that the people have seen, that it looks like magic, perform a few miracles—and then disappear, and for another year nothing happens. The people still have dirty water, no transportation, and no means to make a living. How healthy have they become?"

I was chastened, but the full impact of what she said only came three years later, when I went on a medical mission with a different organization, three months after the 2010 earthquake in Haiti. I came as close to emotional collapse as I had ever been in my life: people bathing in the streets between heaps of rubble and trash, entire neighborhoods flattened as if by an atomic bomb, and fields of people sleeping outdoors because they were too afraid to be inside the suspect buildings that still stood. I slept in a tent with a two optometrists, one of them a Haitian-born man who had moved to the US as a child, and the man's 17-year-old son, coming "home" with his dad for the first time in years to see a ruined land.

It was late April. We spent the first half of every night awake, waiting for it to cool down enough to sleep, and the second half lying awake because of the loud crowing of the fighting roosters penned up 50 feet away from us and the shouts of the men cheering on the cockfights.

More sleep-deprived than in internship or basic training, we went to set up clinic each morning at what was presumably a hospital and nursing school. By the time we arrived, the courtyard would be teeming with people desperate to be seen by the American doctors. We had to press our way inside, and as soon as we did, lines would form to follow us in, three, four or even five people across, clamoring for the chance to be first, or next, or to bypass whoever was in front of them.

The heat and humidity mounted, and the insufficiency of our resources—basic pain relievers, a few simple antibiotics, some rudimentary diabetes medications—became clear. One woman had clearly suffered a debilitating stroke—months ago, probably before "the event." Another was fairly obviously dying of a cancer that even in the US would have been terminal, but here she couldn't even reasonably expect palliative pain medication, since had we attempted to bring any in it would have been confiscated. Scores of people with chronic, manageable diseases got a month's worth of medications to keep their illnesses at bay—until they ran out, and there was no one there to replace them.

I lasted four days, not even staying the full week I had planned. On my last afternoon there, a few of the other participants and I attended a WHO cluster meeting, at which we were cautioned that the prevalence of bleeding stomach ulcers was very high in this area, and most people in the population probably couldn't tolerate treatment with anti-inflammatory pain relievers, like ibuprofen and naproxen—two of the three most common meds we had distributed that week. Ruth Messinger had been completely right—how healthy had I made the people I came to help? I left the WHO meeting thinking I had done nothing but make everyone sicker—including myself.

This would be an awful story if it ended there, but while I was completely out of my element, my colleagues on this trip were not. They were making the first trip of what was to be a long-haul commitment, including a plan to help rebuild that nursing school, improve the training of the local nurses, and build a children's school in the area. There was even talk over dinner one night of trying to build a pharmaceutical plant in the area, to create jobs and supply those people with diabetes, high blood pressure, and treatable skin infections with cheap, locally made versions of the medicines they needed.

Their plan, and my brief, disastrous involvement with it, made me realize that however good I might become at building meaningful, healing relationships with my patients, those relationships cannot happen at all, or at least cannot effect complete healing, if we don't ensure that there is a safe space in which they can exist. Not a "safe space" like the ones being debated on college campuses. In my "safe space," there will *definitely* be uncomfortable topics discussed, and cherished beliefs being challenged. I mean a safe space that guarantees I can have a genuine relationship with a person seeking my help, without conflict of interest, and without outside forces making it impossible for them to carry out the plans we make together.

This means that a connection to the "non-medical" parts of the wider world is essential. In residency, I heard a talk from pediatrician Herb Needleman, whose work on childhood lead poisoning was instrumental in the removal of lead from gasoline and paint in the US—and nearly cost him his career, due to the backlash he faced from the lead industry.

During the talk, he remembered one of the first cases of lead poisoning he saw as a resident at St. Christopher's Children's Hospital in Philadelphia. "I had made the diagnosis and was rather pleased with myself. I knew from what the child's mother had said that he had eaten some chips of peeling paint. So, I strode into the room and said, 'Your child has lead poisoning. We can treat him, but you have to move out of that house. It's contaminated.' And that mom knew a lot more than I did, because she shot back, 'Where should we go? All the houses in our neighborhood are just as bad.'" His treatment was useless, unless the basic facts of this family's life could be changed.

Needleman's legacy runs deep in pediatricians. Lead poisoning is far less prevalent than it used to be, but it's not gone. Within the past year I needed to install lead-safe water filters in my own hundred-year-old house in Pittsburgh because the city still has lead service lines. Children in Flint, Michigan have spent most of the past several years first unable and then afraid to drink the water in their homes due to lead contamination caused by a "cost-saving" measure by the city of Flint and the state of Michigan, one which will end up *costing* millions of dollars and thousands of irreparably damaged lives.

Who brought this crisis to the public eye? Not a politician. A pediatrician, Mona Hanna-Attisha, who knew she couldn't help her affected patients one-by-one in her office, without sounding the alarm to everyone.

Ironically, lead poisoning may count as "low-hanging fruit," when it comes to issues where doctors try to make change in the world. Think about the crises that affected just the patients I saw in one afternoon last week: addiction, domestic violence, inadequate social support for the elderly and disabled, war, persecution, poverty, hazardous work environments, and under-recognition of mental health as health. Trying to approach health and wellness in the world we live in is like fighting a hydra—chop off one head, and two grow in its place.

No one in their right mind would expect one doctor, or even all of medicine together, to solve all of society's problems, or even one of them. Needleman's and Hanna-Attisha's examples, however, demonstrate the possibility of focused action that can actually make a lot of people better over the long run—just like my friend who helped create the possibility of a safe space in the US for people being persecuted due to their sexual orientation. We all have some recurring issue that we find vexing in our practice of medicine. We can complain about it incessantly, or resolve to do something about it.

Nine years ago, my group went out and recruited 40 other community pediatricians and family doctors, and together, we convinced several of our local private schools to close loopholes in their vaccination policies. Last year it was the buprenorphine program, so that our patients struggling with addiction, and others in the community where we practice, could access treatment for their disease and a comprehensive approach to their mental health, chronic pain, and social struggles. What's next on the horizon? Maybe, a senior day care with culturally appropriate food and activities for the elders in our immigrant population, whose family members often can't work because they are home providing care. Who knows?

Maybe, the next step is change that begins at home, with the healthcare system itself. As much as outside crises stand in the way of my patients' wellness, they are a fact of life—they are the reason medicine is needed in the first place, to heal the hurts that the world inflicts. But, if the system itself is getting in the way of healing, by fracturing communication, incentivizing volume of care over quality outcomes, or turning human beings in pain into consumers as if they were buying televisions, that's pretty poor medicine.

I think of my electronic medical record. I hated paper charts, whether it was having to read cryptic handwriting or locate missing pages that turned out to be in a bunker in the Laurel Mountains. On the other hand, is it an advance to have an electronic version, in which the record-keeping function is back-engineered onto what is essentially a program for billing, so that the entire structure of the note is designed to capture "data points" that will increase the "complexity" of the visit—and ends up producing notes that have no syntax, let alone a soul? What good is Meaningful Use, a program to increase the use of the electronic record for tracking referrals, identifying smokers, and reminding us to do screening exams, if the records themselves are meaningless?

Furthermore, it's not the specific product we use. I've used three different EHRs in residency and practice, and all feel like they are directly interfering in how I express myself. I long for a generation of medical records that is narrative—that, when I open a patient's chart, tells me a story about the patient much like he might tell himself, almost as if I am reading a medical memoir.

I think of my schedule, with its 15-minute blocks, even if I sometimes have the luxury of 30 minutes with some patients. There has been research in the last 10 years that has gone so far as to call the 15-minute visit "inhumane" and suggest that it actually perpetuates and exacerbates health disparities in our society. It goes without saying that things are even worse elsewhere in the world. The people I met in Haiti were lucky to get five minutes—any longer and they and I would both have been trampled by the next people in line. Where in this schedule can I both do all of the essential tasks of patient care and conversation we discussed earlier in the book—and find time to make all the "investments" I discussed in this chapter? Who can change the world, or change someone's life, when there is barely time to change the paper on the exam table?

Personally, I'm lucky—the time pressure in my office comes from the nurses and patients, clamoring for more timely, more urgent visits. I am booked, because people are asking for my attention. As such, when I decide to take a longer time for someone who needs it, it is only my next patient with whom I have to negotiate (or grovel). My colleagues in the for-profit world (whether or not their employers acknowledge their profit motive) are seeing more patients, because doing so generates more revenue.

Something needs to change in the payment structure to actually encourage us to invest the time—especially as fewer and fewer physicians are self-employed in a way that would make them able to buck the system and just say, "I'm going to take as long as I need." On the other hand, when we've tried to do this, it seems to backfire. We've seen experiments like "capitation," which essentially turned into rationing, because it gave primary doctors a lump sum of money per patient and said, "Make it stretch as far as you can." Spend too much, and it eats into your own salary. That might cut down on too many unnecessary tests. At some point, however, it also tempted doctors into skipping more expensive tests or treatments that were necessary.

Other experiments, like urgent care or virtual visits, increase accessibility to doctors—but at the expense of continuity, or actually being examined by the doctor. While these visits may be convenient, they are still volume-driven—and all come with the disclaimer that they are not a replacement for a longitudinal relationship with a primary care doctor.

The problem may be that we have tried to graft together too many pieces that don't fit. The cottage industry of family doctors, the academic medical schools, the civic institutions of community hospitals, the technocratic pharmaceutical and medical device industry, and the risk-averse insurers are all trying to coexist in one Frankenstein monster of a system. Whenever it becomes clear that the mix is too dangerous (1906, when the Food and Drug Administration was created) or that too many people are locked out of the system altogether (1965, when Medicare was created, or 2010, when the Affordable Care Act passed), government becomes yet another clumsy, uneasy partner in the alliance. Each actor has its own interests and tries to tilt the balance in a direction that will favor those interests—whether that be more people buying the drugs, or lower insurance payouts, or more places to conduct research studies, even if the research might be slightly tainted by corporate money. Missing from these negotiations? The patients themselves.

No wonder, then, that people keep suggesting that we blow the whole thing up and start over. I got an e-mail a couple years ago from a patient about Direct Primary Care; now it seems like I hear about DPC nearly every day. There are many similar models under names like concierge practice, or Ideal Medical Care. All promote easy accessibility, ongoing relationships, integrated care, with ancillary services often under one roof, and, in many cases, supersede health insurance, because patients are working on a subscription fee, either a monthly or yearly payment to be a "member" of the practice.

One Oregon physician, Pamela Wible, started her Ideal Medical Practice by putting the patients completely in charge. She held a town hall meeting, where she said, "Write my job description. I want to be your doctor. I wanna work for you." Once they were done designing the doctor, they designed the clinic and the way it ran. Wible's mission in her clinic? To humanize medicine, both for the patients, and for herself, a once-burnt-out physician, whose own advocacy centers around preventing physician suicides.

My life would certainly be easier in such a practice, and I'm sure my patients would be more satisfied. But, how many patients could I serve? What would I say to the others who couldn't fit into my 20-hour-per-week schedule of one hour visits? Whom else would they go to—and what kind of care would they get there?

The truth is that these are first-world problems. Even an uninsured, undocumented person in the United States today stands a decent chance of being pulled back from the brink of death in an emergency. However poorly we do, there is a reason even wealthy patients from other countries are seeking care here and not at home, to say nothing of what poorer patients long for when they hope for one of those mirage-like medical missions to deliver them some hope.

However frustrating it is to work in the field of medicine in the United States, something must be luring in the hundreds and thousands of foreign physicians who come here, put their careers on hold *for the chance to be paid and live like a resident*, so many in fact that the US physician shortage is creating a "brain-drain" on the healthcare systems of other countries, who desperately need their physicians. As one new patient told me the other day, "I didn't go to doctors back home—you could say hello to them in the street and before you knew it, they'd have given you a shot and asked you for money." We seem to have the greenest grass around, even if it is full of weeds and bare spots. When people feel that they are nowhere, we are the somewhere they dream of being.

On the other hand, healthcare, and the way we deliver it, isn't a first-world endeavor. It happens everywhere—anywhere there are human beings. The story of the old woman who put me next to God started halfway around the world, as did the story I had you imagine yourself in at the beginning of this chapter. My own story of healing took me to Israel and to Haiti. Marty's story, in Chapter 4, never took him outside of Pittsburgh, while my inveterate smoker in Chapter 8 started life under communism.

In all of those places, medicine begins as a simple transaction. You are human. Even in sickness, even on the brink of death, even when your abilities are severely curtailed, you are human. When you are ill, however, your ability to express that humanity—to *feel* human—is diminished. You come to me, and we form a covenant, in which we promise each other that we will do what it takes to give you complete healing, body and soul, and make you whole again.

The hard part of the transaction is replicating that healing seven billion times, especially in a place where the healer is as close to nowhere as the patient.

Sometimes, a patient will say to me, "You're the only one who listens to me." I'm their medical home, but the rest of the medical neighborhood may as well be boarded up. I am the only one they feel they can come to for compassion and attentive listening, and I am the one who needs to advocate for them to be treated like a person. They may have been profiled as an addict, a belligerent patient, or a hypochondriac, and now that label follows them everywhere. The label may even come from the story I or one of my colleagues chose to put in the medical records. As such, that label means that even if they have pneumonia, or a broken leg, or some other obviously serious diagnosis, they get treated as though they are drug-seeking, or crazy.

If I accept the label, I have given up. The other day I said to my students, "Even if someone has done something awful, committed a crime or something, that's not the *only* thing they've ever done. How many of us have never done something 'bad?' See the whole picture, not just the label."

However, if I'm the only one who stands by them, if I become the one place where all the people who have been labeled and stereotyped can go for help, and I need to advocate for them to get humane treatment every time they go somewhere else in the system, how long can I keep it up? How can I draw boundaries that leave me available to them, while avoiding the burnout my friend Jack asked me about?

The good news is I'm *not* the only one. I can see the compassion and humanity in my colleagues, too. In some, it is obvious, like the people I have the privilege to team with every day in my practice. In some, it needs to be awakened.

The night before I finished this manuscript, I went to hear the brilliant Irish singer-songwriter Glen Hansard in concert. Toward the end of the show, Glen looked out into the audience and said, "Is young Connor here? Connor, do you know this song? Would you like to sing it with me?" A boy of about 10, the same age as my son, came nervously onto the stage and sat timidly next to Glen, a thick curtain of yellow blond hair covering his right eye, and sang. He was in heaven.

About halfway through the song, Connor brushed back his hair for a split second and in doing so revealed that the eye it had hidden from view was misshapen, lower on his face than the other and tilted awkwardly. I felt a twinge of recognition: I had passed him in the restroom earlier, and felt a sort of sadness at the sight of this boy, who looked thin, pale, and out of place.

Now, however, watching Glen play off of him the same way he had done with the other musicians in the band, smiling at him and repositioning the microphone so Connor could be heard, the sadness was gone. Glen's embrace of the boy wiped all that away and replaced it with being able to see who he really was—a budding young musician in his own right, whose mother was the pianist in the ensemble. He was a

10-year-old boy from Ireland who loved music and was enjoying the gift of touring America with a brilliant singer.

One of us, just one healer who is willing to put a different label on someone who is marginalized, can change the system. Daring to label someone as human, as worthy of caring, and sharing that opinion with colleagues is contagious. It can make them see below the surface and find the person in the addict or the human being in the angry, difficult patient. I know this is true, because when I have nearly exhausted myself doing exactly this, it has actually worked. I have seen opinions and attitudes change. It isn't sufficient on its own to rebuild the whole system, but it is the foundation of a whole new system. In that new system, every patient's encounter looks like this:

A 34-year-old woman from Idaho presents today with her husband, having been married and childless for seven years. It has led to much distress in their marriage and a rift between the couple and the husband's parents, who have been very persistent in asking why they do not have children. What I love about *them* is that despite their infertility, they have remained visibly in love and devoted to each other. What I love about my *job* is that I have made it a point of learning this.

Based on the woman's history of irregular periods and deep, hoarse voice, I believe she has polycystic ovarian syndrome. I explain carefully to her that this is a hormonal problem that is not her own fault, and that simple, effective treatments exist. I do so, without once looking at the clock or rushing my explanation, because I refuse to confuse.

I ask my medical assistant with the perfect aim to draw blood to test blood sugar and testosterone levels. There are plenty of other things I could order as well, but my pre-test probability for this diagnosis is so high that I don't feel like it's worth wasting the money or getting unneeded false positive results on some other test. If my diagnosis is correct, we will try treating her with twice-daily metformin and encouragement to enjoy each other's intimate company, in hopes of helping her and her husband conceive the child they have always wanted. If my diagnosis is incorrect, I will take 20 minutes out of my day and either make a phone call or sit down face to face with them to tell them how sorry I am and how frustrated I am with them that we still don't have an answer—and refuse to abandon them.

A year from now, she will return to this same room and say, "Of course, David is coming to see you as his pediatrician. A year ago, you stood here in this room and told me that everything would be fine, and you couldn't wait to see my baby in a year's time. I wouldn't go anywhere else." And I will immediately find him a spot in my schedule.

Healing People, Not Patients

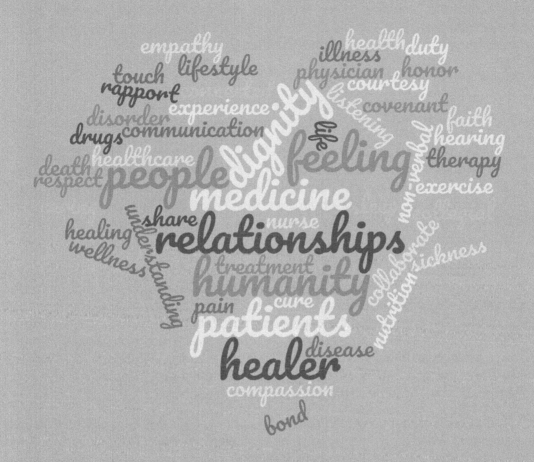

APPENDIX

Being a Nice Jewish Doctor

What follows is a discussion of the Jewish roots for how I approach medicine. As the main text points out, many of the concepts here are part of a common "trunk" to the tree of faith that highlight the respect we need to have for our fellow humans. Nevertheless, the "tree bark" is very important, and sharing my "bark" with you is part of the reason I wrote this book, for the light I think these sources bring to all of us, whether we grew up under my tree or another.

It is not good for God to be alone.

I know, God says, "It is not good for Man to be alone" (Genesis 2:18), but God's actions tell us that God abhors loneliness as well, as unfit for a Divine Being as it is for a human being.

The mystics believe that before creation, God was infinite, all-encompassing, and alone. To make a space in which the universe could come into being, God contracted, shrank, and made space into which another could enter. The beginning of God creating heaven and earth was God making room, humbling so that the otherness could expand and fill the resulting void.

But, not just any Other would do. Light and dark, air and water, land and sea, sun and moon, birds and fish, beasts and vermin were not enough to populate the emptiness. God needed a counterpart, perhaps not an equal, but someone who could strive to keep up. "Let Us," God proposed to the angels, "make human beings in Our image, after Our likeness" (Genesis 1:26). And the angels, the obsequious, sycophantic angels, who had no will of their own, had a fit. They argued, with some saying, "Go ahead—humanity will be kind and loving, humanity will be righteous." The others said, "Stop! Humanity will be liars! Humanity will be in perpetual conflict!" (Genesis Rabbah 8:5).

And in spite of that danger, in spite of the potential for evil, God went ahead with the program. What drove the building of the Golem in the 1500s? What motivated Dr. Frankenstein? Why did the humans in *Battlestar Galactica* build Cylons that would eventually annihilate them? As much as we see the dramatic irony in those stories, we cannot but look at Genesis and wonder, "Didn't God know what was coming?" The answer, of course, is that God knew. God always knows. And God did anyway.

But, what was this "image" in which God created humans? God had no body, only an infinite mind. Melvin Konner writes, "… this Johnny-come-lately people … tell the world's great civilizations that you shouldn't carve or hammer an image of a god … worship *only* a body-less, invisible, unitary god. An abstraction … A disembodied voice booming out of a cloud or bush. A ghostly, forceful, collective memory. An all-knowing, all-seeing, all-thinking mind, with a capital M if you like, but a mind only" (Melvin Konner, *The Jewish Body*, 2009). Fragments of that mind are believed to have dispersed though the universe at the moment of *tzimtzum*, contraction, that brought the void into existence. The vessels that held the divine essence shattered and scattered across the cosmos. A world, yet to be created, was, in a sense, already broken. How could God, deliberately self-limiting so that existence could happen, put it back together, without swallowing everything back up.

Healing People, Not Patients

With a partner, of course, one who could team with God in bringing the world into the kind of existence that God intended all along. A partner of the world, and yet also of God, at the same time. So, God gathered dust from the four corners of the earth, and instilled it with something unique, something that none of the animals were given: God's own breath (Genesis 2:7). One Hebrew word, *neshima*, signifies breath; change the vowel to *neshama*, and it becomes the word for soul, or living human being. A living being so precious that to destroy it is as if one has destroyed the entire world; to save it is like saving the entire world (Mishna Sanhedrin, 4:5).

With that partner, God forms a covenant—many covenants, actually, sealing the promises with symbols like rainbows (Genesis 9:13), circumcision (Genesis 17:10), and stone tablets engraved with the law (Exodus 24:12). The essence of the Jewish faith, the place where a Jew's worth as a person is tested most thoroughly, is in the relationship with God—and the parallel relationship with other human beings made in God's image.

Decades ago, Rabbi Harold Schulweis wrote that the relationship between physician and patient is likewise one of covenant, "two persons, aware of each other's humanity" (Schulweis, "The Doctor in the Patient"). Schulweis points out that the myths of twentieth century medicine, in which the patient is helpless and the doctor omnipotent, are tearing the healing relationship apart. But, what if healing breaks free of those myths? Then, the real healing can begin, healing where there is a "dialogue of trust" and where doctor and patient "struggle in common against pain and disease."

Schulweis' comment places the medical relationship, the one which defines so much of my life, in the context of what my teacher's teacher, Rabbi Brad Artson, has said: "To love someone is to become vulnerable to his or her choices" (Artson, "On the Way—A Presentation of Process Theology"). For God, the same God who sacrificed infinitude in order to contract and make room for a universe, this means that God is inextricably invested and bound up in what we humans are doing. God is with us in our suffering, feels our pain, suffers our losses.

Are we physicians then supposed to liken ourselves to God? Surely we've been accused often enough of doing that anyway.

Truth be told, we *are* supposed to liken ourselves to God. God didn't create us in the physical image of the Divine, for there is no such thing. We walk after God's ways, do what God does, imitate God's performance of acts of loving-kindness (Talmud Tractate Sotah, 14a). Among these is the act of visiting the sick, an act capable of restoring the soul of one who is in despair of ever being whole again (Ozarowsky, *To Walk In God's Ways*). This act of merely visiting the sick, to say nothing of actually providing medicine, is so powerful that it can take away one-sixtieth part of the suffering of the person who is ill, provided the visitor is a *ben gilo*, a kindred spirit in whom the patient can see himself reflected (Kestenbaum, "The Gift of Healing Relationship").

Our mission as doctors, even before we apply the stethoscope, or write a prescription, is to be that *ben gilo*, to find our commonality with the person across from us. But, medicine, healing and curing disease, is also in the realm of God's acts of loving-kindness. God is the original cardiologist and the first wound care nurse, "the healer of broken hearts, and the one who binds their wounds" (Psalm 147:3). We merely follow in those footsteps.

As for the swagger in our step while we retrace those footsteps, the prophet Micah reminds us, "do justice, love mercy, and walk *humbly* with your God" (6:8).

Anyone who has visited with the sick, especially if they are not a physician, knows the awkward silences that ensue. We are don't visit in order to talk, but to listen. When people suffer, God listens, just as God listened to the Israelites in Egypt, crying out in their suffering (Exodus 3:7). When people suffer illness, those who sit with them listen attentively, if they really wish to be of help. Just as the Israelites were strangers in Egypt when God heard their cries, we encounter people in their illness who are strangers as well. They no longer recognize their bodies, have lost the ability to make familiar, unthinking movements, or perhaps cannot even rely on their minds.

Others are not just estranged from themselves, but from the world at large. There are no fewer than 36 commandments and exhortations in the Torah not to wrong the stranger (Talmud Bava Metzia 59b), beginning with Exodus 22:20: "Do not wrong a stranger, and do not oppress him, because you were strangers in Egypt." Nachmanides explains that God means, "I behold the tears of such who are oppressed and have no comforter, and on the side of their oppressors there is power, and I deliver each one from him that is too strong for him." Rashbam looks particularly at the commandment not to oppress and understands, "he has no 'redeemer' who looks out for his interest. G'd mentioned this to remind the Israelites who also had no one in Egypt to plead their case."

Rabbi Jonathan Sacks, former Chief Rabbi of the British Commonwealth, points out that even when Joseph was vizier to Pharoah, before the enslavement, his Egyptian servants did not dine with Joseph's brothers, "because Egyptians could not eat with Hebrews, for that is detestable to Egyptians." In contrast, Sacks reasons, the Israelites are commanded to treat the stranger fairly, "because you know the soul of the stranger (Exodus 23:9)"—out of empathy.

The Mekhilta follows these sources and reasons that the stranger is actually greater than the Jew: "Now who is greater? One who loves the King or one whom the King loves? Certainly, one whom the King loves." No surprise, then, that Sacks concludes, "the most serious offence—for the prophets as well as the Mosaic books—was the use of power against the powerless: the widow, the orphan and, above all, the stranger."

It is easy to be a *ben gilo* to someone who is like you and to take away his suffering. To really walk humbly with God requires making yourself into a *ben gilo* for someone who is not like you—to set aside differences, see beyond barriers, and find a commonality. The magic of being created in the Divine Image is that God is "as close to us as breathing, and as far as the farthermost star" (*Gates of Prayer*). Even as God is unfathomable and unreachable, God looks at us as if looking in a mirror. How much closer we are to one another than any of us is to God. Consequently, how much easier it should be to see ourselves reflected in each other's faces.

You wouldn't spit at your own face in the mirror, or call it names, or slander it, or murder it. You would value someone who held a piece of your own soul in them as highly as you did yourself. This is what the commandment to "Love your neighbor as yourself (Leviticus 19:18)" means, the commandment which Rabbi Akiva held to be the greatest principle in the whole Torah (Jerusalem Talmud Nedarim 30b:1). A person's dignity, possessions, life itself should be as dear to you as your own (Mishna Avot 2:10). If their blood is being shed you may not stand idly by (Leviticus 19:16), even if that blood is actually their money (the words are similar in Hebrew) or even their time, which is being wasted or stolen.

Blood, however, can be shed in bloodless ways. Hurtful words, ones that shame a person so badly that their face goes pale, are like committing murder (Rashi on Leviticus 19:17). Accordingly, even when criticizing a sinner, we have to watch our words (multiple commentators on the same verse, and Talmud Tractate Arachin 16a). As healers, we have the privilege and the hazard of speaking to people about some of the most sensitive subjects there are: sex, obesity, drug abuse, unemployment, aging, and dying. It used to be believed that the High Priest in the Holy of Holies could destroy the world, if he had but one impure thought; in the same way, one misplaced word from a doctor, even an unintended or misinterpreted one, can crumble a patient's entire world.

Furthermore, we do not operate in a vacuum. We are intertwined in our profession with countless other professionals, functionaries, clerks, and technicians. Each has the duty to heal, to greet everyone with a bright face and judge everyone favorably (Mishna Avot 1:6, 1:15), and when even one of us fails, "they shall stumble one upon another, as it were before the sword, when none pursueth" (Leviticus 26:37). The commentary to the verse from Leviticus says that all Israelites are each other's guarantors, but it's true of any group, where those outside the group identify all the members with one another, under a single label. The group stands or falls together (Talmud Shevuot 39a and Sanhedrin 27b).

What are these duties that each of us carries? Not to curse, or label, or denigrate those for whom we care. Not to place the enforcement of the rules ahead of the achievement of healing. And, not to withdraw into ourselves and restrict our involvement in the enterprise to "just doing our jobs."

Hillel the Elder said, "If I am not for myself, who will be for me? But, if I am for myself alone, what am I? And if not now, when (Avot 1:14)?" Only I can carry out those responsibilities that are mine; no one else will do them for me. But, if I only stick to "just doing my job," what good am I to the people I am supposed to help? In fact, am I even really doing my job, if I carry out the minutiae at the expense of the overall goal? And, why am I waiting for someone to give me permission to do it, when either the same outcome will happen in 10 minutes, or the entire matter will be forgotten when "something important comes up," and I will have done nothing at all to help this person.

Psychiatrist Rabbi Abraham Twerski, for decades a leader in the fields of self-help and recovery from addiction, suggests that perhaps, "If I am not for myself" means that one who only exists as defined by others, or by what he does for others, has a poor self-concept (*Visions of the Fathers*). For a healthcare employee who feels that they are on the bottom rung of the ladder, that poor self-concept can come out at the worst possible moments, whenever their good intentions are thwarted, and they are made to feel inferior or unworthy. This could mean being brushed off by a specialist, put on hold by an insurer, or told by an equally well-meaning colleague that this particular martyr's mission will need to wait until their desk is cleared of other tasks.

This balance between self-importance and self-sacrifice is essential to the functioning of the healthcare system. One of the early Chasidic masters had a tradition of carrying two slips of paper, one in each pocket. On one he wrote: 'for my sake, the world was created.' On the other he wrote: 'I am but dust and ashes.' He would take out each slip of paper as necessary, as a reminder to himself.

Of this tradition, Rabbi Toba Spitzer suggests, "Dive into the pocket of 'for my sake was the world created.' This pocket reminds us that we are all created in the image of God. It is a reminder that as children of the first human, our inheritance is all the blessings of Creation. This world is here for us, too" (Toba Spitzer, "Two Pockets"). Without this remembrance of our own divine nature, we may forget that of those around us—first our colleagues, and eventually our patients. While we need the "dust and ashes" pocket to keep us humble enough to remember that we are fallible, and that we must often subjugate our needs to those of others in order to recognize their divinity, it is by keeping in mind our own resemblance to God that we fashion around us a culture that does justice to our ideals.

In that culture, we dispense a medicine that goes beyond the technically advanced, but soulless, medicine that is the hallmark of much of Western medical practice today. While deeply respecting the scientific advances of our time, we strive to provide care that goes beyond the technical. We spoke of loving-kindness, and the relationship of our brand of medicine is like the relationship of loving-kindness to charity (Talmud Tractate Sukkah 49b; needless to say, the analogy to medical practice is mine).

Charity, teaches the Talmud, can be achieved only with money. So, it is true that only antibiotics can cure pneumonia, and only surgery can remove a tumor obstructing the bowel. Technical medicine is like money. Loving-kindness, however, can be achieved with either money or with personal involvement. At 11:30 at night on a long call in my third year of medical school, the senior resident on my surgery team sat (sat!) on the bedside of our first surgery patient for the next morning. He gave a peptalk about how well he expected the surgery to go and answered questions. All the while, he ignored the impatient intern who was pacing the hallway, waiting until our team could go get a snack. He was investing of himself in the man's well-being. This is medical loving-kindness.

Charity can be given only to those who are poor. One must be ill, in poor health, actually have a tumor or infection to benefit from the wonders of the technical cures for these ills. On the other hand, what if one only fears illness? The loving-kindness of patiently standing by a patient, until those fears can be quieted, can benefit even the rich, even when they do not know they are rich with good health. Even those in the full bloom of good health benefit from our presence, from our keen interest in their lives, from working to identify possible sources of pain or discord that could disrupt that flowering, and address those problems before they surface.

Charity can be given only to those who are alive. Loving-kindness can be bestowed upon the dead and the dying and those who survive the dead. When all of our technology has failed to extend live beyond the years that God grants us, our loving-kindness can make the last days of a dying man peaceful and meaningful, his passing painless, and his family whole by providing comfort and closure that our machines cannot do.

Fashioning such a culture is a daunting task, an uphill battle that has been the project of Judaism for 3,500 years. Can a handful, or even an army, of well-meaning doctors, nurses, pharmacists, and patients in the 21st century CE possibly do what has not been done until now?

There is a saying in Mishna Avot quoted so often it is almost trite. "He (Rabbi Tarfon) used to say: It is not your responsibility to finish the work, but neither are you free to desist from it" (2:16). But, the previous verse is less well known:

"The day is short and the work is much, the workers are lazy and the reward is great, and the Master of the House is pressing" (2:15).

A mere 15 minutes with 90 minutes of work to do saps our desire to do anything at all, except stick to the script. The work, however, is so much, because of the great reward, the chance to preserve, prolong, and improve human lives, and interact with Divine souls every minute of the way. The Master of the House is pressing, and so are the countless souls, created in His image, who need our help. They do not need us to finish the work, for they would not be able to wait that long even so. They need us now. And if not now, when?

empathy
illness health duty
touch lifestyle physician honor
rapport courtesy
experience dignity covenant
disorder listening faith
drugs communication life feeling hearing
healthcare non-verbal therapy
death people medicine exercise
respect
share nurse
healing understanding relationships collaborate sickness
wellness treatment
humanity nutrition
pain cure
patients
disease
healer
compassion
bond

NOTES

❏ Chapter 1:

- The Kurt Vonnegut quotation is from his "Address to Graduating Class at Bennington College, 1970."

- GOMER is an acronym meaning "Get Out of My Emergency Room," applied to elderly patients with intractable medical problems and dementia in the farcical novel *The House of God*, written by Samuel Shem.

- "Shake and bake" refers to a cancer patient with fever and neutropenia. I borrowed it from the play *Wit*, by Margaret Edson, where it is used flippantly by Jason Posner, an oncology fellow who is more comfortable in the lab than in a patient's room.

- "Status hispanicus" is taken from Danielle Ofri's *What Doctors Feel*, and is a term used by many of her residency classmates to describe a hysterical patient screaming nonsensically in Spanish about a problem they believe is blown out of proportion. I do not endorse the use of any of these terms, but they do require explanation.

- For a discussion of the idea of humanism in medicine, see the website of the Arnold P. Gold Foundation at http://www.gold-foundation.org/.

- The Maslach Burnout Inventory can be found in numerous places online, including http://www.fresno.ucsf.edu/wellness/documents/MaslachBurnout.pdf.

- The discussion of the Exodus and its importance to understanding individual suffering comes from Rabbi Irving Greenberg's article "Judaism as an Exodus Religion."

- *To Walk In God's Ways* is by Rabbi Joseph Ozarowsky. Ozarowsky tells the story of the great Rabbi Akiva personally visiting a student and restoring him to health by tending to his home while the student is ill.

- "The Second Sentence," by Jonathan Kole, appeared in *Annals of Internal Medicine* in 2014.

- Reb Aryeh Levine's quotation about his wife's feet is referenced in *Jewish Wisdom*, by Rabbi Joseph Telushkin.

❏ Chapter 2:

- The six basic things all doctors need to know refer to the core competencies, and can be explored in greater detail in the Common Program Requirements of the Accreditation Council on Graduate Medical Education (ACGME), available at http://www.acgme.org/acgmeweb/Portals/0/PFAssets/ProgramRequirements/CPRs_07012015.pdf

- "Worst-case scenario thinking," "rule outs," and other cognitive errors that interfere with doctors' attention their patients' stories are discussed in Leana Wen and Joshua Kosowsky's book, *When Doctors Don't Listen: How to Avoid Misdiagnoses and Unnecessary Tests*.

- Adam Wright and colleagues conducted the 2010 interview with Lawrence Weed in the *Journal of the American Medical Informatics Society*, "Bringing science to medicine: an interview with Larry Weed, inventor of the problem-oriented medical record."

- I do not have a source for the folktale of the boy reciting the alphabet. I first heard it in elementary school, the same school my children now attend. I imagine they, too, will hear this story there. However, the idea of using attentive listening skills to "put the letters together" parallels the discipline of *Narrative Medicine*, described in detail by Rita Charon in her book of the same title. Charon writes, "The altruistic listener listens to advance the project of the authentic speaker so that, after a while, the speaker says, 'Thank you, now I understand what I meant to say.'"

❑ Chapter 3:

- Much of the discussion of using questions to uncover real meaning, instead of factoids, is based on the idea of differentiating the experience of illness from the biological disease. For the best-known articulation of this idea, read The Illness Narratives: Suffering, Healing and the Human Condition, by psychiatrist Arthur Kleinman. Like me, Kleinman worked extensively with refugees, many of them through the Harvard Refugee Trauma Program. The set of questions he developed, often called "the Kleinman questions," attempt to uncover the deeper layers of meaning that patients and cultures ascribe to illnesses.

- Kosowsky's exercise "No Questions Asked" is also described in *When Doctors Don't Listen*. His observations on that exercise, including the relative usefulness of different ways of asking questions, were part of a quantum leap for me in how I approach a conversation with a patient.

- The study on mothers measuring fever "qualitatively" by placing a hand on a forehead, was one that I was taught as gospel in residency, but for which I do not remember the source. It was our way of reassuring ourselves that we knew better.

- Data on languages in the world are from www.linguisticsociety.org. The information on where the handful of specific languages mentioned are spoken is information I learned myself from the speakers of those languages I have met over the years, and the translators I was fortunate enough to find.

- The work of Abraham Verghese and colleagues on the Stanford 25 is available online at www.stanfordmedicine25.stanford.edu.

- "Naked" first appeared in the *New England Journal of Medicine* in 2005 and later in Gawande's book *Better*.

❑ Chapter 4:

- I might never have begun this project had I not read Bernard Lown's book *The Lost Art of Healing* in the summer of 2000. Two chapters of that book, "Words that Maim" and "Words that Heal," made me keenly aware of the power of the words I speak in the clinical encounter. The sense I have made of the stories in this chapter is thanks to the lessons I learned from reading Lown's book.

- The story of the Cascadia tsunami is from *The New Yorker* from July 20, 2015. A similar description of how Native American "data" is ignored, and why it shouldn't be, is the basis of Lori Arviso Alvord's book, *The Scalpel and the Silver Bear*, about her experiences becoming and practicing as the first Navajo woman surgeon. Alvord's journey culminates in learning to reintegrate her native heritage into a fuller understanding of how to heal those she cares for.

- Marty Makary's chapter on a physician called The Raptor in *Unaccountable: What Hospitals Won't Tell You and How Transparency Can Revolutionize Health Care* features an excellent discussion on the ways in which physicians verbally abuse patients.

- For a discussion of motivating through fear, refer both to *The Lost Art of Healing*, and to Otis Brawley's book, *How We Do Harm*, in which he discusses the use of the fear of cancer to drive increased use of testing and pursuit of treatment in prostate cancer and other malignancies.

- Gilbert Welch's observations of diagnosing "pre-disease" and the harm it causes are in his book, *Overdiagnosed*.

- My discussion of motivational interviewing draws from Theresa Moyer's article, "The Relationship in Motivational Interviewing," published in *Psychotherapy* in 2014.

- The discussion of finding the right balance of words, and actions, at end of life is informed by the works of multiple authors. Timothy Quill wrote an article which was formative for me about the first and last time he ever said, "There's nothing more we can do for you" to one of his patients. I have been unable to locate the source on repeated attempts. Other material in this section draws on Nicholas Christakis' work *Death Foretold*, Michael Stein's *The Lonely Patient*, and an article by Anthony Back and colleagues called "Abandonment at the end of life from patient, caregiver, nurse, and physician perspectives: loss of continuity and lack of closure."

- Speaking of closure, the program materials are online at www.closure.org.

❏ Chapter 5:

- The story of the resident and her white coat is in the anthology *On Becoming a Doctor*, a creative non-fiction volume edited by Lee Gutkind.

- My research on perceptions of white coats and preferences of physician dress included articles by Amir Kazory, Anna Cha, and colleagues; S. Menachem and P. Shvartzman; S. Sundeep and K.D. Allen; and Shakib Raiman and colleagues. Full citations for each article are in the bibliography and reference section. The idea of dress-down days is addressed at length by Fred Lee in *If Disney Ran Your Hospital: 9 ½ Things You Would Do Differently*.

- Gawande's "Naked" and work by Catherine Wellberry underpin my discussion of patient dress including the indignity of gowns.

❏ Chapter 6:

- Fred Lee's book provided important food for thought for this chapter as well, discussing the role of front line employees, including the need to empower them to step outside the strict rules in service of the patient's needs. Makary also discusses workplace culture, using some of the same examples as Lee, in *Unaccountable*.

- The concept of lost lifetime comes from advocate Laura Casey, in her book *How to Get the Healthcare You Want: The Savvy Consumer's Guide to Navigating the Health Care System*.
- "Hotspotting" is described in another of Atul Gawande's *New Yorker* articles, and is a project of Dr. Jeffrey Brenner at Camden Health. A fuller description is online at http://hotspotting.camdenhealth.org/.
- Discussions and definitions of the Patient Centered Medical Home are available at https://pcmh.ahrq.gov/page/defining-pcmh. Those interested in the process of becoming a medical home should read the blog of Dr. Fred Peltzmann at http://www.medpagetoday.com/PatientCenteredMedicalHome/.

❑ Chapter 7:

- The story of the Rohingya is summarized in Esther Htusan's article "Lack of health care deadly for Burma's Rohingya" in *The Washington Post*, May 8, 2014. https://www.washingtonpost.com/world/lack-of-health-care-deadly-for-burmas-rohingya/2014/05/08/ac5a9ae8-d6e6-11e3-8a78-8fe50322a72c_story.html.
- A sobering account of the role of race in American medicine, and especially in the city of Atlanta, is in Otis Brawley's and Paul Goldberger's book, *How We Do Harm: A Doctor Breaks Ranks About Neing Sick in America*. The article on undertreatment of pain in African-American children is my MK Goyal and colleagues and is entitled, "Racial Disparities in Pain Management of Children With Appendicitis in Emergency Departments." It ran in *JAMA Pediatrics* in 2015.
- The concept of Lifeworld was developed by Elliot Mishler, a colleague of Arthur Kleinman's at Harvard. My source on the topic is "Giving Voice to the Lifeworld. More Humane, More Effective Medical Care? A Qualitative Study of Doctor-Patient Communication in General Practice," by C.A. Barry and colleagues.
- Atul Gawande, in addition to discussing hotspotting and immodestly dressed patients, has written on the medicalization of old age in *Being Mortal*. He pays particular attention to the shift in focus between life being meaningful and life being "safe" as people age.
- Those interested in the topic of mental health advance directives can find more information here: http://www.mentalhealthamerica.net/psychiatric-advance-directives-taking-charge-your-care.
- Arthur Kleinman's *Illness Narratives* details the marginalization of gay patients and HIV positive persons in multiple different chapters. Kleinman's discussion of the idea of stigma, including the origins of the term and how different illnesses become stigmatized in different societies, is fundamental to my understanding of how these patients are treated.

❑ Chapter 8:

- Danielle Ofri's *What Doctors Feel* contains a stark description of Joanna, an ED physician who becomes increasingly jaded towards patients such as those described in this chapter. Her anger at them ultimately leads her to develop her own addictive behavior, to alcohol, and eventually to ruin her medical career.

- The WHO data on worldwide mortality comes from WHO Fact Sheet No. 310, "The Leading Causes of Death," available online at http://www.who.int/mediacentre/factsheets/fs310/en/.

- The relative costs of cardiac catheterization vs. counseling to quit smoking come from a 2013 column in the *New York Times* blog, "Well" (http://well.blogs.nytimes.com/2013/08/15/heart-stents-continue-to-be-overused/?_r=0) and from the American Academy of Pediatrics website at https://www2.aap.org/richmondcenter/pdfs/PACTReimbursementforSmokingCessation.pdf. The numbers for tobacco counseling are somewhat out of date but they highlight the low reimbursement and lack of universal coverage for the labor-intensive, low-tech interventions involved.

- Links to the original Surgeon General report from 1964 and later related materials is online at www.whyquit.com. This includes the discussion of the difference between using habit vs. addiction language when talking about smoking. I do not recall the name of the lecturer whose findings I reference in the text, but numerous patients have validated his premise for me; all agree that there is a part of their brain that understands exactly how to quit and another part that routinely sabotages the whole thing.

- Michael Moss wrote the 2013 article in the *New York Times Magazine* entitled, "The Extraordinary Science of Junk Food," which elucidates concepts like the bliss point, the advertising strategies used by the food industry, and the approach to opening new markets that occasioned Jeffrey Dunn's remark about Coke in Brazil.

- The statistics about food deserts in Pittsburgh, as well as some of the conceptual definitions, are from Zachary Murray's report, "A Menu for Food Justice: Strategies for Improving Access to Healthy Foods in Allegheny County," published in 2013 by the local advocacy group Just Harvest.

❏ Chapter 9:

- The statistics on how long it would take to deliver appropriate primary care come from RAND researcher and former Pitt Med faculty member Ateev Merhotra, and from Fred Pelzmann's blog referenced above.

- The discussion of pre-operative clearance references guidelines for this process published in 2014 by the Anesthesiological Society of America. These are available online through PubMed.

❏ Chapter 10:

- If you are a medical provider and the description of the patient in Chapter 10 sounds unfamiliar, it is because this doesn't describe one disease, but rather a cluster of disturbing symptoms that affects numerous middle-aged and older patients in one of the refugee populations for which I care. It is a syndrome that cries out for a better approach to medicine, precisely because it does not fit into any of the boxes in the current system and requires a lot of communication, time, and compassion.

- The description of the narrative process in writing parallel notes on patients comes from Rita Charon's *Narrative Medicine*.

- There is a growing literature on Balint groups. This section relies on "Compassion fatigue and burnout: the role of Balint groups" by J. Benson and K. Magraith, and on "Research on Balint groups: A literature review" by K. Van Roy and colleagues.

- The literature debunking Andrew Wakefield's study on the MMR vaccine is vast. Those who are interested in a succinct, two-part explanation of the issues can visit the Khan Academy online for their videos tracing the history of the problem. The statistic regarding mortality gains is a rough estimate and is attributed to my teacher Dr. Don Middleton, who in first year lecture was quick to point out how vast the gains of public health (vaccines and sanitation) were compared to all the modern medical technology combined.

- Oncotalk resources are online at http://depts.washington.edu/oncotalk/. Back, Arnold, and Tulsky's book *Mastering Communication with Seriously Ill Patients* contains a longer discussion of the same techniques and includes exercises for the clinicians eager to trial the techniques in the office. "That Dragon Cancer" was profiled on National Public Radio and in *Wired* magazine in early 2016 (http://www.wired.com/2016/01/that-dragon-cancer/).

- Links regarding the various alternate delivery systems, including Ideal Medical Care, concierge practice, and comprehensive primary care plus follow here:
  - ✓ http://www.npr.org/sections/health-shots/2016/01/13/462898517/can-concierge-medical-care-work-for-the-middle-class
  - ✓ http://www.idealmedicalcare.org/blog/
  - ✓ http://www.idealmedicalcare.org/blog/how-to-be-the-doctor-you-always-wanted-to-be-explicit-language/
  - ✓ https://innovation.cms.gov/initiatives/comprehensive primary-care-plus/
  - ✓ http://www.politico.com/agenda/story/2016/04/obamacare-delivery-reform-000088

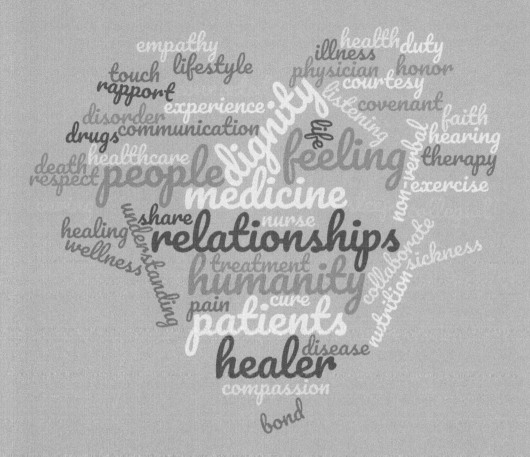

REFERENCES AND
SUGGESTED RESOURCES

10 Tips for Working with Transgender Individuals. San Francisco: Transgender Law Center, 2011.

Albert SM. Jewish Teachings on Family Caregiving Responsibility (oral presentation). Beth Shalom Congregation, Pittsburgh, PA. January 24, 2015.

Alvord LA, Van Pelt EC. *The Scalpel and the Silver Bear: The First Navajo Woman Surgeon Combines Western Medicine and Traditional Healing*. New York: Bantam, 1999.

Back A, Arnold R, Tulsky J. *Mastering Communication with Seriously Ill Patients*. New York: Cambridge University Press, 2009.

Back A, Young J, McCown E, Engelberg R, Vig E, Reinke L, et al. Abandonment at the end of life from patient, caregiver, nurse, and physician perspectives: loss of continuity and lack of closure. *Arch Intern Med* 2009;169(5):474-479.

Barry CA, et al. Giving voice to the lifeworld. More humane, more effective medical care? A qualitative study of doctor-patient communication in general practice. *Soc Sci Med* 2001;53(4):487-505.

Berger Z. *Talking to Your Doctor: A Patient's Guide to Communication in the Exam Room and Beyond*. Lanham, MD: Rowman and Littlefield, 2013.

Bleier CS, Donnelly L, Granowitz SP. *L'Chaim: To Good Health and Life. A History of Montefiore Hospital of Pittsburgh, Pennsylvania* 1898-1990. Pittsburgh, PA: Bleier, Donnely, and Granowitz, 1997.

Brawley O. *How We Do Harm: A Doctor Breaks Ranks About Being Sick in America*. New York: St. Martin's Press, 2012.

Casey LL. *How to Get the Health Care You Want: The Savvy Consumer's Guide to Navigating the Health Care System*. Austin, TX: 1 Life Press, 2007.

Cha A, et al. Resident physician attire: does it make a difference to our patients? *Am J Obstet Gynecol* 2004;190(5):1484-1488.

Charon R. *Narrative Medicine: Honoring the Stories of Illness*. New York: Oxford University Press, 2006.

Charon R, Herrmann N. A sense of story, or why teach reflective writing? *Acad Med* 2012 Jan; 87(1):5-7.

Christakis N. *Death Foretold: Prophecy and Prognosis in Medical Care*. Chicago: University of Chicago Press, 1999.

Dyche L, Swiderski D. The effect of physician solicitation approaches on ability to identify patient concerns. *J Gen Intern Med* 2005;20:267-270.

Edson M. *W;t*. New York: Faber and Faber, 1993.

Egnew TR, et al. Integrating communication training into a required family medicine clerkship. *Acad Med* 2004;79:737-743.

Fadiman A. *The Spirit Catches You and You Fall Down: A Hmong Child, Her American Doctors, and the Collision of Two Cultures*. New York: Farrar, Strauss, and Giroux, 1997.

Fiscella K, Epstein RM. So much to do, so little time: care for the socially disadvantaged and the 15-minute visit. *Arch Intern Med* 2008 September 22;168(17):1843-1852.

Gawande A. *Better: A Surgeon's Notes on Performance*. New York: Picador, 2007.

-----. *Complications: A Surgeon's Notes on an Imperfect Science*. New York: Picador, 2002.

Goyal MK, et al. Racial disparities in pain management of children with appendicitis in emergency departments. *JAMA Pediatr* Online First: September 14, 2015.

Greenberg I. Judaism is an Exodus religion. *Living the Holidays*. New York: Summit Books, 1988.

Groopman J. *How Doctors Think*. Boston: Houghton Mifflin, 2007.

-----. *The Anatomy of Hope: How People Prevail in the Face of Illness*. New York: Random House, 2003.

Gutkind L (ed). *Rage & Reconciliation: Inspiring a Health Care Revolution. Creative Nonfiction*, Volume 21.

----. *Silence Kills: Speaking Out and Saving Lives*. Dallas: Southern Methodist University Press, 2007.

Halevi Y (translation by Cole P). Where Will I Find You? *Poetry Magazine*. http://www.poetryfoundation.org/poetrymagazine/poem/243646

Helman CG. Disease versus illness in general practice. *J R Coll Gen Pract* 1981;31:548-552.

Hofstadter D. Ant fugue. *Escher, Godel, Bach: An Eternal Golden Braid*. New York: Basic Books, 1979, 1999:311-336.

Htusan E. Lack of health care deadly for Burma's Rohingya. *Washington Post*. May 8, 2014 https://www.washingtonpost.com/world/lack-of-health-care-deadly-for-burmas-rohingya/2014/05/08/ac5a9ae8-d6e6-11e3 8a78-8fe50322a72c_story.html

Jauhar S. *Intern: A Doctor's Initiation*. New York: Farrar, Strauss, and Giroux, 2008.

Kazory A. Physicians, their appearance, and the white coat. *Am J Med* 2008 Sep;121(9):825-828.

Klass P. *Treatment Kind and Fair: Letters to a Young Doctor*. New York: Basic Books, 2007.

Kleinman A. *The Illness Narratives: Suffering, Healing, and the Human Condition*. New York: Basic Books, 1988.

Konner M. *The Jewish Body*. New York: Schocken, 2009.

Lazare A. *On Apology*. New York: Oxford University Press, 2004.

Leanza Y, Boivin I, Rosenberg E. Interruptions and resistance: a comparison of medical consultations with family and trained interpreters. *Soc Sci Med* 2010;70(12):1888-1895.

Learning styles: all students are created equally (and differently). Teach.com. http://teach.com/what/teachers-teach/learning-styles

Lee F. *If Disney Ran Your Hospital: 9 ½ Things You Would Do Differently*. Bozeman, MT: Second River Healthcare Press, 2004.

Lown B. *The Lost Art of Healing*. Boston: Houghton Mifflin, 1996.

Makary M. *Unaccountable: What Hospitals Won't Tell You and How Transparency Can Revolutionize Health Care*. New York: Bloomsbury Press, 2012.

Manning K. Reflections of a Grady Doctor. http://www.gradydoctor.com/

Meier L (ed). *Jewish Values in Health and Medicine*. Lanham, MD: University Press of America, 1991.

Menahem S, Shvartzman P. Is our appearance important to our patients? *Fam Pract* 1998;15(5):391-397.

Moss M. The extraordinary science of addictive junk food. *New York Times Magazine*. February 20, 2013.

Moyers TB. The relationship in motivational interviewing. *Psychotherapy* 2014;51(3):358-363.

Mullan F. Me and the system: the personal essay and health policy. *Health Aff* 1999 Jul/Aug;18(4):118-124.

Murray Z. *A Menu for Food Justice: Strategies for Improving Access to Healthy Foods in Allegheny County*. Pittsburgh, PA: Just Harvest, 2013. http://www.justharvest.org/jh_publication/a-menu-for-food-justice-strategies-for-improving-access-to-healthy-foods-in-allegheny-county/

Naisbitt J, Naisbitt N, Phillips D. *High Tech, High Touch*. New York: Broadway Books, 1999.

O'Connor A. Heart stents still overused, experts say. "Well" blog. *New York Times*. August 15, 2013. http://well.blogs.nytimes.com/2013/08/15/heart-stents-continue-to-be-overused/?_r=0

Ofri D. http://danielleofri.com/

-----. *Singular Intimacies: Becoming a Doctor at Bellevue*. Boston: Beacon Press, 2003.

-----. *What Doctors Feel: How Emotions Affect the Practice of Medicine*. Boston: Beacon Press, 2013.

Ozarowski JS. *To Walk in God's Ways: Jewish Pastoral Perspectives on Illness and Bereavement*. Northvale, NJ: Jason Aronson, 1995.

Pelzman F. Starting a journey: building a new model of care. Building the Patient-Centered Medical Home. June 13, 2013. http://www.medpagetoday.com/PatientCenteredMedicalHome/PatientCenteredMedicalHome/39813

-----. Getting the phone to stop ringing. Building the Patient-Centered Medical Home. August 27, 2015. http://www.medpagetoday.com/PatientCenteredMedicalHome/PatientCenteredMedicalHome/53274

Polito JR. The Surgeon General's Reports: 50 years of cessation ignorance. WhyQuit News. http://whyquit.com/pr/012014.html

Quill T, Cassell C. Nonabandonment: a central obligation for physicians. *Ann Intern Med* 1995;122:368-374.

Rehman SU, et al. What to wear today? Effect of doctor's attire on the trust and confidence of patients. *Am J Med* 2005;118:1279-1286.

Rhoades DR, et al. Speaking and interruptions during primary care office visits. *Fam Med* 2001 Jul-Aug;33(7):528-532.

Schultz K. The really big one. *New Yorker*. July 20, 2015. http://www.newyorker.com/magazine/2015/07/20/the-really-big-one

Sefaria. www.sefaria.org*

Shelton A. *Transforming Burnout: A Simple Guide to Self-Renewal*. Tacoma, WA: Vibrant Press, 2007.

Shem S. *The House of God*. New York: Putnam, 1978.

Smedley BD, Stith AY, Nelson AR (eds). *Unequal Treatment: Confronting Racial and Ethnic Disparities in Health Care*. Washington DC: National Academies Press, 2003.

Smedslund G, Berg RC, Hammerstrøm KT, et al. Motivational interviewing for substance abuse. *Cochrane Database Syst Rev*. 2011; :CD008063.

Spiro H, McCrea Churnen MG, Peschel E, St. James D (eds). *Empathy and the Practice of Medicine: Beyond Pills and the Scalpel*. New Haven, CT: Yale University, 1993.

Spitzer T. Two pockets. *Kol Nidre* (Yom Kippur) sermon 5771. 2010. http://dorsheitzedek.org/writings/two-pockets

Stanford Medicine 25. Stanford Medicine Department of Medicine http://medicine.stanford.edu/residency/stanford-25.html

Stein M. *The Lonely Patient: How We Experience Illness*. New York: William Morrow, 2007.

Stepanyan KD. On losing your humanity. *Ann Intern Med* 2015;163:479-480.

Street RL, et al. How does communication heal? Pathways linking clinician-patient communication to health outcomes. *Patient Educ Couns* 2009;74(3):295-301.

Teeter BS, Kavookjian J. Telephone-based motivational interviewing for medication adherence: a systematic review. *Transl Behav Med* 2014;4(4):372-381.

Telushkin J. *A Code of Jewish Ethics, Volume 1: You Shall Be Holy*. New York: Bell Tower, 2006.

---

*Extensive collection of Jewish texts including Bible, Talmud, commentaries, legal codes, ethical texts, prayerbooks, etc. Texts are available in Hebrew and English and cross-linked to allow for deep study or compilation of resource sheets. Specific texts relevant to this book are cited parenthetically in the appendix.

-----. *Jewish Literacy*. New York: William Morrow, 1991.

The top 10 causes of death. WHO Fact Sheet No. 310. http://www.who.int/mediacentre/factsheets/fs310/en/

Transue E. *Patient by Patient: Lessons in Love, Loss, Hope, and Healing from a Doctor's Practice*. New York: St. Martin's Griffin, 2008.

Twerski A. *Visions of the Fathers*. Brooklyn, NY: Shaar Press, 1999.

Tyson P. The Hippocratic Oath today. NOVA. http://www.pbs.org/wgbh/nova/body/hippocratic-oath-today.html

UpToDate. www.uptodateonline.com

Wear D, Varley JD. Rituals of verification: the role of simulation in developing and evaluating empathic communication. *Patient Educ Couns* 2008;71(2):153-156.

Weinberg RB. Communion. *Ann Intern Med* 1995;123(10):804-805.

Welch HG, Schwartz LM, Woloshin S. *Overdiagnosed: Making People Sick in the Pursuit of Health*. Boston: Beacon Press, 2011.

Wellbery C, Chan M. White coat, patient gown. *Med Humanit* 2014;40:90-96.

Wen L. The Doctor Is Listening: An E.R. Physician Writes About What You Need to Do to Get the Best Health Care Possible. http://whendoctorsdontlisten.blogspot.com/

Wen L, Kosowsky JM. *When Doctors Don't Listen: How to Avoid Misdiagnoses and Unnecessary Tests*. New York: St. Martin's Press, 2012.

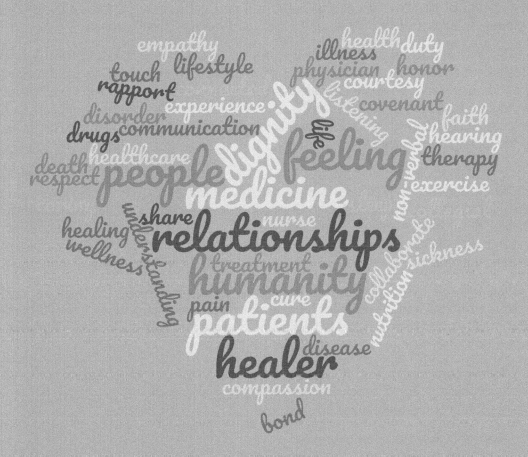

ABOUT THE AUTHOR

Jonathan Weinkle, MD, FAAP, is a general internist and general who came to medicine after deciding against careers as a philosopher or a rabbi. He practices primary care medicine at a busy urban community health center, providing comprehensive care to patients of all ages with and without insurance, representing a broad diversity of languages, faiths, cultures, native lands, and socioeconomic backgrounds.

Dr. Weinkle also serves as a medical advisor to the *Closure* project of the Jewish Healthcare Foundation, a program intended to improve the quality of care and change the individual experience at end-of-life. Also under the auspices of the JHF, he is crafting a program to help clinicians master the core competency of respectful communication with patients and families, based largely on the concepts, principles, and ideas detailed in this book and the research underlying it.

In addition, Dr. Weinkle serves as Clinical Assistant Professor in the Departments of Pediatrics and Family Medicine at the University of Pittsburgh (his *alma mater*), and as medical director of the Physician Assistant Studies Program at Chatham University. Driving all of these endeavors is a strong commitment to infusing his interactions with patients with the core values of his Jewish faith, beginning with the idea that both patient and provider are created in the Divine image and must act and be treated accordingly.

Dr. Weinkle lives with his wife and three sons within blocks of both his own childhood home and his mother's. Furthermore, if he ever gets a long enough break from all the things listed in this bio, he plans to record a singer-songwriter album that taps into the same core ideas as his career and teaching.

Follow Jonathan online at www.healerswholisten.com or on social media at @ healerswholisten. For questions regarding speaking engagements, programming, etc., please contact media@healerswholisten.com.

Website: www.healerswholisten.com
Facebook: www.facebook.com/healerswholisten
Twitter: @healerswholistn
Instagram: @healerswholisten